IS ST...   ...J?

- Do you suffer from insomnia?

- Do you feel anxious for no particular reason?

- Would you like to feel better about your life?

- Have you had trouble keeping your weight under control?

- Do you hate the idea of taking prescription drugs for depression?

ST. JOHN'S WORT: THE MIRACLE HERB MAY BE JUST THE HELP YOU NEED

MICHAEL E. THASE, M.D., is a professor of Psychiatry, Medical and Research Director, Mood Disorders Module, and Associate Director, Clinical Research Center, Department of Psychiatry at the University of Pittsburgh School of Medicine, Western Psychiatric Institute and Clinic, Pittsburgh, Pennsylvania.

ELIZABETH E. LOREDO works as an editor in the publishing group of an educational television company and has written a wide range of nonfiction books, as well as magazine articles. She lives in New York City.

ST. JOHN'S WORT:
Nature's Mood Booster

MICHAEL E. THASE, M.D. & ELIZABETH E. LOREDO

AVON BOOKS ◆ NEW YORK

The ideas, procedures, and suggestions in this book are intended to supplement, not replace, the medical advice of a trained medical professional. All matters regarding your health require medical supervision. Consult your physician before adopting the suggestions in this book, as well as about any condition that may require diagnosis or medical attention. The authors and publisher disclaim any liability arising directly or indirectly from the use of this book.

AVON BOOKS, INC.
1350 Avenue of the Americas
New York, New York 10019

Copyright © 1998 by CMD Publishing, a division of Current Medical Directions, Inc.
Published by arrangement with CMD Publishing, a division of Current Medical Directions, Inc.
Illustrations by Patricia Shea
Visit our website at **http://www.AvonBooks.com**
Library of Congress Catalog Card Number: 98-92452
ISBN: 0-380-80288-0

First Avon Books Printing: August 1998

AVON TRADEMARK REG. U.S. PAT. OFF. AND IN OTHER COUNTRIES, MARCA REGISTRADA, HECHO EN U.S.A.

Printed in the U.S.A.

WCD   10   9   8   7   6   5   4   3   2   1

Contents

ONE

What Is St. John's Wort?

St. John's wort doth charm all the witches away.
If gathered at midnight on the saint's holy day.
And devils and witches have no power to harm
Those that do gather the plant for a charm:
Rub the lintels and post with that red
  juicy flower
No thunder nor tempest will then have the power
To hurt or to hinder your houses: and bind
Round your neck a charm of a similar kind.

Vickery, A. R. 1981. "Traditional uses and
folklore of Hypericum in the British Isles,"
Economic Botany vol. 35: 289–295

Perhaps one of the elements most disturbing to doctors about herb-based remedies is the fact that so many of their patients begin treatment with them without knowing even the most basic facts about the herbs. That's certainly been the case with St. John's Wort as with others that have benefited from the blinding but brief media spotlight. When I first began researching this book, I asked a number of people, a few of them patients, what they knew about St. John's Wort. Virtually everyone recalled hearing something like "it works on depression"—some even excitedly described it as "a miracle drug" for the condition. Most people knew it was an herb or "some kind of plant." But when pressed for details not one could muster anything more, nor answer even the most rudimentary questions about the herb's history, actions, or applications. Yet many I spoke with had already recommended St. John's Wort to friends suffering from depression, and a few were even using it themselves.

That kind of casual dosing may sound absurdly reckless, but is put into perspective when you recall how often patients take away a scribbled prescription from a doctor, fill it, and use the entire sample without being able to even name the drug they've taken. Patients often can't say when or how to take a medication they've been prescribed until they can read the abbreviated instructions the pharmacist has printed on the label. Yet many patients will blithely continue taking other medications without the least idea that doing so might be rendering the new prescription useless or even harmful—because they never learned their various medications posed a conflict. This is all information patients should have before stepping one foot from the doctor's office.

Some doctors expect their patients to volunteer information about medications they are taking for conditions being treated by other doctors, while patients figure their doctor would initiate a discussion on side effects or drug conflicts if there was anything to be concerned about. Both should accept the responsibility for sharing this kind of information, but because this is not a perfect world, that doesn't usually happen. Patients are often too anxious or timid to volunteer any such information, if they even recall it under the strain many people feel while visiting physicians of any kind. Too many physicians are therefore not aware of factors in their patients' lives that might make certain medications—herbal or prescription—an unpleasant or dangerous option. Doctors sometimes do not have the time or inclination to take the updated histories that would alert the team to potential problems. Other times, physicians will consciously withhold information, in perhaps misguided efforts to prevent the power of suggestion from amplifying a drug's possible actions or side effects (i.e., a "negative" example of the placebo effect). They err by not providing enough information to guide patients through uncomfortable or frightening symptoms. And, even when patients feel they are not getting enough information, they have trouble asking, "What exactly *is* this?"

Now, when you combine that kind of unquestioning faith with the inherent belief many people share that anything "natural" can't be bad, you can get a dangerous cocktail in terms of medicinal effects. People hear from a trusted friend, media source, or ad that an herbal remedy will have such-and-such action. And that's enough. "What harm could it do?" is the prevailing attitude.

But that's precisely the question. What harm *could* an herbal remedy do? Don't be fooled—herbal treatments like St. John's Wort, when used for medicinal purposes, should be handled with the same caution as prescription drugs. When it comes right down to it, finding out the answer is up to you. Ask questions. Learn the basics of any medication you use in your treatment so that you have the tools to find out even more. Probe for information on what's in your medication, where it comes from, what it's reported to do. That will help you understand what it's doing for you in terms of physical and mental changes, good or bad, while you're taking it. So, because the best place to start your herbal "homework" is at the beginning, this first chapter provides a basic primer on the plant itself. It will serve as a brief introduction to St. John's Wort— tracing the herb's family tree, and probing for facts about its chemical makeup. Armed with this information, you should find it easier to make sense out of the research-study results and jargon that inevitably accompany explorations of any medical treatment. These facts also will help shed light on the role of St. John's Wort in depression therapy as well as the many other uses with which the herb is credited. But first you'll learn a little of the long history and intriguing mythology surrounding St. John's Wort, which indicate that the herb is no novelty drug however new it may seem now that it is being hawked in ads and health-food stores. In the current renaissance of herbals, St. John's Wort is a perfect case study of the old adage "everything old is new again."

What is Saint John's Wort?

Saint John's Wort is an herb. In fact, St. John's Wort's very name defines it—"wort" means plant or herb in Old English. Technically, an herb is any plant known to have medicinal or culinary uses—St. John's Wort has both those properties. It can be tossed into salads as a slightly bitter green, but of course that's not what's causing all the excitement. It's the healing action that St. John's Wort is claimed to have, on

depression and literally dozens of other conditions, that is gar-
nering the attention.

Who first discovered the medicinal uses of St. John's Wort? A bunch of monks?

St. John's Wort has an incredibly long history as a medicinal herb, predating Christianity, Buddhism, and the monastery
gardens of their monks. What we know of the herb's early use
as a medicine we discover in ancient pharmacopoeias—books
listing therapeutic plants and their habitats, actions, uses, preparation, dosages, and cautions. St. John's Wort appears in
some of the oldest surviving pharmacopoeias, written in
Greece and Rome over 2,000 years ago. The herb was undoubtedly used for many years prior to those first written records, as they were merely collections of medical lore already
well-known at the time—there are Asian and Egyptian herbals
and pharmacopoeias far more ancient. However, for the first
records documenting St. John's Wort, we rely on the works
of Hippocrates and Pliny. Hippocrates was a Greek physician
living around 400 B.C., whose groundbreaking practice of
healing-as-art has since earned him the title "the Father of
Medicine." A holistic physician, Hippocrates wrote "to heal
even an eye, one must heal the head, and indeed the whole
body." This approach involved the careful prescription of certain herbs—"let your medicine be your food and your food,
medicine"—used in combination with other treatments. St.
John's Wort numbered among the limited list of herbs Hippocrates recommended.

Pliny, a Roman scholar in the first century A.D., further explored the use of herbals, and included St. John's Wort in his
list of prescribed remedies. At about the same time, St. John's
Wort also made an appearance in the *De Materia Medica*, a
5-book treatise on medicinal therapies derived from plants,
animals, and minerals written by Pedanius Dioscorides. Dioscorides was a Greek physician who observed the use of St.
John's Wort while serving as a surgeon to the Roman army
around A.D. 78. He noted the herb's effects upon the sword
gashes and spear-puncture wounds he dressed on the battle-
field. His documentation of 500 plants and their actions
became the definitive resource on the subject. Astonishingly,
his work wasn't significantly improved upon until the

Renaissance—after a period of almost 1,600 years appropriately called the "Dark Ages." That means St. John's Wort was in constant use by physicians during that extended period, too.

Galen was another noted Greek physician who prescribed St. John's Wort in his work; his writings appeared in the second century and enlarged on the old Greek idea that all ailments arose from changes in the body's fluids. Galen categorized these fluids and what he believed to be their effects into 4 groups called "humors": blood (producing bad temper), phlegm (sluggishness), black bile (melancholy) and yellow bile (irritability). It was his contention that the varying combinations of these 4 types of fluids determined a person's unique state of health and temperament. He prescribed St. John's Wort for the treatment of many ailments presumed to be brought on by disturbances of these 4 humors.

Herbalism next experienced an explosion in the 1500s, as exploration expanded borders and many more plants were "discovered" by European herbalists. Remedies were exchanged between cultures, and the first botanic gardens were planted for study in Italy. In Switzerland, a man named Paracelsus incorporated this abundant new knowledge into a new theory of medicine. Paracelsus believed that the very appearance of a plant suggested its medicinal actions. In fact, his Doctrine of Signatures asserted that you could determine what conditions a plant might treat by its shape—the plant would resemble the body parts targeted by the diseases it could be used to prevent or cure. In Paracelsus's Doctrine, St. John's Wort's bright gold color indicated it would be helpful in the treatment of liver conditions, like jaundice, or choleric conditions such as gastritis. Paracelsus also deduced that the herb could be used to stop hemorrhaging from puncture wounds or cuts, because the oil glands in the leaves of St. John's Wort resembled punctures and the oil flowed bloodred when released. This doctrine was well accepted for many years and was actually required reading in medical schools at the time!

Ironically, Paracelsus's work on St. John's Wort also marked the beginning of the plant remedy's slow slide into temporary obscurity. Paracelsus included chemical-based medicines in his writings, and these later came to replace plants as the therapies of choice, largely because they tend to be more easily synthesized into commercial drugs than are plants.

Culpeper's Herbal followed on the footsteps of Paracelsus. Inspired by the earlier Doctrine, Nicholas Culpeper produced his own work in the early 1600s. Defying tradition, he wrote his book in easy-to-read English rather than the Latin physicians had been using in pharmacopoeias to safeguard their medical secrets. Although it caused an angry sensation in medical circles, it was enormously popular among laymen. The *Herbal* is still the book many herbalists reach for today—in chain stores, it's shelved right beside this year's newest books. John Parkinson's *Theatre Of Plants*, also published in the 1600s, was another definitive text. Books like these finally replaced Dioscorides's *Materia Medica*, which had been the herbalist's "bible" for well over a millennium. St. John's Wort is featured in all of them.

The practice of healing was one of great importance in early cultures, considered in the nature of a religious rite. This tradition underwent a slight shift during the Middle Ages, when the use of herbal remedies passed from the wise women of the village and wandering physicians to the monks tending monastery gardens. Monks initially prescribed remedies in combination with a doctrine of faith healing. During this period, written documentation of herb use became more common, since monks were more apt to be literate and compile records. St. John's Wort was used by these medieval monks mainly as a salve for wounds and for bronchial problems involving the throat and lungs, although its effects on melancholy and mania were also noted at the time.

Because of its popularity and broad range of uses, St. John's Wort was a shoo-in when the first botanic garden in the U.S. was designed in the early 1700s by the "Botanizer Royal for America," John Bartram. In fact, St. John's Wort was one of the inaugural herbs planted there. However, Native Americans were already using it to reduce fevers, stop the flow of blood from wounds, as a balm for the skin, and as an antidote for snakebites. But after some initial popularity, St. John's Wort was not mentioned in many subsequent American pharmacopoeias. Its days as a primary medication were soon numbered in any case, both here and abroad, as were those of most herbal remedies, because the next hundred years saw a steady increase in the popularity of made-in-the-pharmacy medications, called chemotherapies (not to be confused with the more common use of that term today).

Why did herbs like St. John's Wort stop being popular? How come everyone doesn't use herbal remedies today?

There were many factors that contributed to the decline in use of herbals. As people moved from agricultural areas and into cities in the seventeenth and eighteenth centuries, they tended to lose the affinity for "home remedies" that had formed the basis of herbal treatments like St. John's Wort. There was a growing desire for modernization in all things, and particularly medicine, which made chemical treatments more appealing. But even before that, herbal therapies were dealt a tremendous blow when literally thousands of herbal practitioners were killed during the Puritan witch-hunts of England, New England, and elsewhere.

Before the advent of synthetic drugs, herbal remedies were very often dispensed to the poor by the region's "wise women," who were sometimes viewed as witches. These women passed their accumulated lore down the generations through word of mouth. For centuries, wise women had been the doctors and therapists of their day, the ones who knew all the herbs growing in the local fields. Better yet, they *knew* their patients, sometimes too intimately. They understood what their neighbors were suffering and usually had a pretty good handle on why, and so could prescribe for the "whole" patient: For example, if village gossip might help them to diagnose melancholy as the cause of lower back pain, they might prescribe St. John's Wort for both its analgesic and nervine effects.

The Puritan Church's relentless pursuit of witches reduced the population of these women and abruptly stopped dissemination of the knowledge they had collected through the generations. When this was followed by the advent of modern chemistry, use of herbal remedies declined steadily. What followed were dark days for herbals. In the eighteenth century St. John's Wort and other herbals became largely relegated to back pantries and dismissed as quackery, along with the tonics of traveling con men. Claims about an herb's healing properties were called old wives' tales. And, of course, that's just what they were. In this case, however, the tale was not based on superstition or fabrication. It would be almost a century before herbs were once again considered a viable option for health care.

I've heard there are a lot of stories about St. John's Wort, not all of them medicinal. Do they have any basis in fact?

While clearly not required reading, it's nonetheless interesting to discover the many myths surrounding an herb. Sometimes they can give scientists clues about a plant's therapeutic properties. There are a number of superstitions governing the use of St. John's Wort. In one, inhabitants of the Isle of Wight claimed a traveler who stepped on the herb after dark risked being carried off by a ghostly horseman. Another medieval myth centered on placing the herb under your pillow; supposedly this would ensure that St. John would feature in your dreams, bestowing blessings to keep you healthy and safe for the coming year. Another story posited that red spots would appear on the herb's flowers on the anniversary of the saint's beheading. The devil and his demons were thought to hate the flowering herb's sunny golden glare, so carrying it was believed to provide protection from Satan. Other pagan superstitions attributed to the herb included an ability to divine whether a marriage would take place or when someone might die, as evidenced in this poem from Germany:

> The young maid stole through the cottage door,
> And blushed as she sought the plant of power.
> Thou silver glow-worm, oh! lend me thy light,
> I must gather the mystic St. John's Wort to-night;
> The wonderful herb whose leaf will decide
> If the coming year shall see me a bride.

Hobbs, Christopher, *Pharmacy in History*

St. John's Wort also served to drive out the devil from any home where it was hung in the doorway. Centuries later, Pennsylvania Dutch farmers would label it "blessed herb" and use it to protect their infants, in the belief that it would ward off the evil eye if hung in the entry of the home of a newborn child. We suspect that such demon-repelling superstitions surrounding St. John's Wort actually reflect the herb's use as a treatment for depression and related emotional difficulties. In the past, those mysterious and misunderstood conditions were thought to be the work of the devil.

I've heard there are different kinds of St. John's Wort. Which one are we talking about?

It's indeed true that St. John's Wort is a name applied to many different plants. They all reside within the same family, but not all seem to work in the same way medicinally. The species upon which this book focuses is that most frequently tested for effects on depression: *Hypericum perforatum L*, abbreviated as *H. perforatum*. Herbalists and scientists refer to the specific species name when working with, reporting on, or purchasing the plant, in order to avoid confusion, but because the name St. John's Wort is the one with which most consumers are familiar, that common name will be used in this book.

Using Botanical and Common Names

Herbs, like other plants, are often given diverse names in different parts of the world—even herbs in adjoining backyards may be called something different by neighboring gardeners. For decorative flowers, this multitude of names is merely confusing, but for potent medicinal herbs such confusion can lead to a frustrating waste of time when treating with the wrong herb—and could be deadly. Enter Carolus Linnaeus (born Carl von Linne), a Swedish botanist living in the 1700s. Linnaeus developed a system of classifying and naming plants, often using their ancient names as the basis for his terminology. The study of this system is called taxonomy: the classification of everything living into families and orders based on their unique and similar characteristics. In the botanical organizing system, plants have a "first name," a genus, which is capitalized. The genus links different plants that share common elements; in the case of St. John's Wort, the genus is *Hypericum*. The "last

continued

name,'' or second name, designating species is written without any capitalization. The specific species of St. John's Wort we'll be discussing is *Hypericum perforatum* (pronounced hi-PEER-uh-cum per-for-AH-tum). Finally, since some botanists disagree about which plants are related, a letter may follow a name, indicating which botanist classified it with that name. Thus, *Hypericum perforatum L,* lets us know that name was assigned by Linnaeus. Remember, when studying or buying herbs, the only way to get exactly what you want is to use this specific botanical name.

What family of plants does St. John's Wort belong to?

Here's what St. John's Wort's extended family tree looks like:

Division: *Magnoliophyta*
Class: *Magnoliopsida*
Subclass: *Dicotyledoneae*
Superorder: *Dilleniidae*
Order: *Theales*
family: *Hypericaceae* aka *Clusiaceae* or *Guttiferae*
sub family: *Hypericoideae*
genus: *Hypericum*
species: *perforatum*

Remember, the topmost "branches" of this family tree are the broadest category of plant; the lower down on the list, the more specific a category it becomes.

Where did the herb get its name?

Which one? There are as many as 39 different folkloric, or common names, for *Hypericum perforatum*. Perhaps half those common names are associated with biblical terms, like the one used in this book—St. John's Wort. Some of the other names include: amber, amber touch and heal, blessed herb, devil's scourge, God's wonder herb, grace of God, goatweed, Herb of Destiny, hundred holes, Klamath weed, Llamath weed, Rosin Rose, and terrestrial sun. The plant has other names in the many places it is grown around the world: In Germany, it is called *Johanniskraut* (translation: John's cabbage or, from Old High German, John's moss), and in Russian it is *Zveroboi*, or beast-killer, which could be a result of the phototoxic effect it can have on grazing cattle or its use to fend off demons.

The modern botanical term for the plant's genus, *Hypericum,* actually comes from one of its more ancient names. Centuries ago, the Greeks called the plant Hyperion, for the Titan father of their sun god, Helios. The word *Hypericum* itself has been given many different interpretations, but the most popular theory is that it is derived from Greek words meaning "over an apparition," probably a reference to the habit of hanging clippings of the herb over religious icons as protection from evil spirits. *Perforatum* comes from the pattern of clear dots made in the leaves by the plant's transparent oil glands. When light shines through these oil pockets, the leaves do give the appearance of being perforated.

Centuries later, pagan religions called the herb by another name, but one which had a similar meaning to *Hypericum*— *Fuga Daemonum,* meaning scare-devil or demon-frightener. When Christianity took hold in Europe, all those ancient names became objectionable. The common name was changed to *Herba Sancti Ionnis,* or St. John's Wort. This was in honor of the first St. John or John the Baptist. The herb has been said to first bloom each year on his birthday, June 24. The red oil that's produced by crushing the leaves has been called a reminder of St. John the Baptist, who was beheaded. Other sources believe the name refers to a second St. John, the patron saint of nurses. These sources suggest that the second St. John used Hypericum on the wounds of knights during the Crusades.

Why is St. John's Wort named after a saint?

St. John's Wort has a long history of just such religious connections, giving some indication of just how valuable it was as a healing plant to many cultures over the centuries. We know a plant is important when it becomes associated with a group's magic, ritual, and religion, particularly those centered around healing or worship of the sun, often a culture's most important deity. The Greeks used the herb in various rituals

in celebration of Helios, father of the sun god Apollo. Teu-
tonics honored Baldur, their version of Apollo, with offerings
of the herb.

Later, in medieval Europe, St. John's Wort was sometimes
prescribed in cases of "possession"—not surprising, given
our new understanding of how it operates on depression,
thought then to be the work of the devil. Pagans burned it in
bonfires celebrating Midsummer's Eve, one of the most important festivals in their culture. St. John's Wort was included
in these ceremonies as an instrument of sun worship and was
thought to appeal to benevolent fairies.

Ancient mythology made much of the small translucent circles in the leaves, formed by the plant's oil glands, likening
them to tiny suns. Throughout history, these pinpricked leaves
and the herb's golden flowers fostered images of light and
enhanced the connection to various sun gods. Of course, when
Christianity eclipsed paganism, such festivities were no longer
acceptable. But the sunlit imagery of St. John's Wort had too
strong an appeal, and its medical effects were too popular to
ignore. Just as the early Christians absorbed Halloween into
their own rituals as a way of attracting former pagans, so too
did they assimilate St. John's Wort. The herb was still prescribed, but under a new common name honoring a Christian
holy man, and so became known as St. John's Wort.

What kind of name *is* "wort" anyway?

Wort is Old English for "plant" and, as noted earlier, the
herb was named in honor of one of the Christian saints. So
the name simply means St. John's plant.

What does St. John's Wort look like?

Many of the various species within the *Hypericum* family
have a very similar appearance. *H. perforatum* is a classic
example of this family "resemblance." The plant can grow as
tall as five feet and has many stems that branch in their upper
parts; the plant can get quite bushy. Each of these branching
stems has very separate and distinct runglike leaves that are
long and round-tipped, usually described botanically as oblong
or elliptical. Each branch ends in the attractive, sunny yellow
flower, appealing enough to be grown as an ornamental. The
flower assumes a star-shaped pattern of 5 petals, lying open

like a pinwheel. You have to look closely to spot the series of tiny black dots ringing the ruffled outer edges of the petals.

The center of each flower has a spherical pistil surrounded by an explosion of 50 or so stamens. Buds are a paler yellow and tightly wound to a sharp point. Flowers occur in clusters, in botanical terms "inflorescences," and typically appear in late June through early fall in the U.S. The bright green leaves are spotted by small translucent oil glands. The effect when held up to the light is to make the leaves seem perforated by myriad holes through which the light shines in tiny, sunlike spots. This effect has been described as giving the leaves a "silver lining," a turn of phrase that may be especially apt when St. John's Wort is helpful as an antidepressant. There are also darker-colored oil glands under the leaves and petals and within the buds that are less apparent, until you crush the leaves in your hand and find it covered in crimson oil.

A Primer on Plant Biology and Sexuality

St. John's Wort is a "perfect flower." Depression sufferers finding relief with the herb would no doubt concur with this sobriquet, but in plant terms what it really means is that St. John's Wort has both stamens and pistils. Stamens are the male organs of the plant—in a St. John's Wort plant, these are the 50-odd slender, spiky stalks crowding in 3 clusters around the heart of the flower. That heart, not surprisingly, is made up of the female organ, or pistil. The pistil holds the ovary, which carries the plant's embryonic seeds. St. John's Wort's pistil sprouts three antenna-like protuberances called styles, themselves topped by stigmas coated with sticky material to capture the pollen needed to fertilize seeds. Because each of its flowers has both male and female organs, St. John's Wort is called a hermaphroditic, or self-impregnating plant.

Does St. John's Wort have a scent?

St. John's Wort is classified as an aromatic, which by its definition means the plant has an aroma, though an aromatic

ST. JOHN'S WORT FLOWER AND FLOWER PARTS

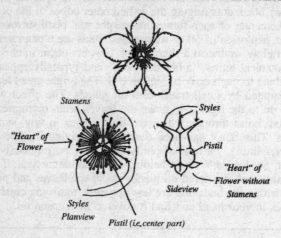

Stamens

"Heart" of
Flower

Styles
Planview

Pistil (i.e, center part)

Styles

Pistil

"Heart" of
Flower without
Stamens

Sideview

could be anything from sweetly appealing to powerfully unpleasant. St. John's Wort's scent is somewhere between those
two extremes. The plant smells mildly medicinal, reminiscent
of turpentine, but with faint lemony undertones.

**What are some of the other species of *Hypericum*? Is it
easy to get them confused in the wild?**

Someone who doesn't spend a lot of time examining plants
would probably have a hard time distinguishing between some
relatives of the 400-odd *Hypericum* species in the wild. Some
grow to much less impressive heights than *Hypericum perforatum*, and some are not branched. A few have more rounded
petals and leaves. But for those people who can't tell a pansy
from a petunia, the differences will seem slight. Many of the
species present a similar, attractive, 5-petaled flower, as well
as the classic small oblong leaves on a branched stem. The
biggest clue to identifying *H. perforatum* is obtained by holding its petals up to the light. Look for the transparent dots
made in the leaves by the plant's oil glands. To my knowledge, no other species within the family shares that trait. Here
are a list of other species:

SPECIES OF HYPERICUM

Note: Many of these plants go under the common name of St. John's Wort. If their common name is known and is different, it is indicated.

SPECIES	COMMON NAME
H. acutum [Synonym of H. tetrapterum]	
H. acutum	
H. aegypticum	
H. anagalloides	Bog St. John's Wort
H. androsaemum	Tutsan (from the French toute-sante, or heal-all)
H. annulatum [Synonym of *H. intermedium*]	
H. barbatum	
H. beanii	
H. brasiliense	
H. buckleii	
H. calycinum	Aaron's Beard, Creeping St. John's Wort
H. canariense	
H. cayennense [Synonym of Vismia cayennensis]	
H. cerastoides [Synonym of H. rhodoppeum]	
H. cernuum Roxb. [Synonym of H. oblongifolium]	
H. chinense [Synonym of H. monogynum]	
H. cistifolium	
H. confertum	
H. coris	
H. crispum [Synonym of H. triquetrifolium]	

H. crux-andreae	St. Peter's Wort
H. cumilicola	Highlands Scrub Hypericum
H. dyeri	
H. elatum [Synonym of H. × inodorum]	
H. erectum	
H. formosum, variety of scouleri	
H. fragile	
H. frondosum	Golden St. John's Wort
H. glandulosum	
H. grandifolium	
H. hircinum	
H. hirsutum	
H. hookeriamnum	
H. hookerianum, var. leschenaultii [Synonym of H. leschenaultii]	
H. hookerianum	
H. humifusum	
H. hypericoides	St. John the Worker, St. Andrew's Cross
H. hyssopifolium	
H. inordorum	
H. intermedium [Synonym of H. annulatum]	
H. japonicum	
H. kalmianum	
H. kamtschaticum, var. senanense [Synonym of H. senanense]	
H. kelleri	
H. kouytchense	
H. lancasteri	
H. lanceolatum	
H. leschenaultii [Synonym of H. hookerianum]	

H. lobocarpum
H. longistylum
H. lysimachioides
H. maculatum
[Synonym of
H. punctatum]
H. monogynum
[Synonym of
H. chinense]
H. montanum
H. montbretii
H. mutilum
H. oblongifolium
H. olympicum
H. orientale
H. patulum   *Kinshibai* (in Japan)
H. perforatum   St. John's Wort, Common
                              St. John's Wort, amber,
                              amber touch and heal,
                              blessed herb, devil's
                              scourge, God's wonder
                              herb, grace of God,
                              goatweed, Herb of
                              Destiny, hundred holes,
                              Klamath weed, Llamath
                              weed, Rosin Rose, and
                              terrestrial sun

H. polyphyllum
H. pratense
H. prolificum   Shrubby St. John's Wort
H. puctatum
H. punctatum [Synonym
    of *H. maculatum*]
H. reflexum f.
H. repens
H. reptans
H. revolutum   Curry Bush
H. rhodoppeum
[Synonym of
H. cerastoides]

H. roeperanum
H. rumeliacum
H. scabrum
H. scouleri
H. senanense
   [Synonym of
   H. kamtschaticum, var.
   senanense]
H. spathulatum
   [Synonym of
   H. prolificum]
H. sphaerocarpum
H. tertrapterum
   [Synonym of *H.
   acutum*]
H. tomentosum
H. triquetrifolium
   [Synonym of *H.
   cuspum*]
H. uralum
H. webbii
   [Synonym of
   H. aegypticum]
H. wilsonii
H. × inodorum
   [Synonym of
   H. hircinum,
   H. androsaemum]
H. × moserianum   Gold Flower
   [Synonym of
   H. calycinum,
   H. patulum]
H. yakusimense

Do the other species work on depression?

H. perforatum is so far the only real contender in this field,
although some other species contain hypericin and pseudo-
hypericins in varying levels. That doesn't mean very much at
the moment, however, since it's not certain that hypericin is
the active ingredient. The other species may not have the pre-

cise combination of hypericin and other active ingredients that will work effectively on depression. Instead, many of the *Hypericum* species are used anecdotally or are being tested for their effects on a variety of other conditions.

Where does the herb grow?

You name it. Those unaware of the potential clinical uses for St. John's Wort would be more apt to classify the herb as a weed, since this hardy plant can be found thriving in almost any patch of dry, sunny ground. Even moderately shady spots can harbor a stand of the herb. It does especially well in uncultivated areas ravaged by logging operations or other kinds of soil disruptions. St. John's Wort also sprouts untended in hedges, meadows, unmown pastures, beside highways, and in the woods. Its easy adaptation to almost any environment in which it's introduced (except the extremes of desert, tropic, and tundra) is one of the reasons St. John's Wort is unflatteringly considered a weed in most parts of the world. It pops up in backyards, empty lots, and in the floral borders of municipal buildings where gardeners are looking for a plant that needs no care. The herb is native to Britain, Europe, and Asia. Though it is not indigenous to North America, St. John's Wort has made a home here—with a vengeance. See the chart below for a list of the places where St. John's Wort has been spotted, and the countries around the world it can be found.

OTHER COUNTRIES WHERE *HYPERICUM PERFORATUM* MAY BE FOUND*

Afghanistan	Gansu, China
Albania	Guizhou, China
Algeria [north]	Hebei, China
Armenia	Henan, China
Austria	Hubei, China
Azerbaijan	Hunan, China
Belarus	Jiangsu, China
Belgium	Jiangxi, China
Bulgaria	Shaanxi, China

*Source: USDA-ARS GRIN Database

Shandong, China
Shanxi, China
Sichuan, China
Xinjiang, China
Cyprus
Czechoslovakia
Denmark
Finland
France [incl. Corsica]
Georgia
Germany
Greece [incl. Crete]
Hungary
India [northwest]
Iran
Iraq
Ireland
Italy [incl. Sardinia, Sicily]
Kazakhstan
Kyrgyzstan
Lebanon
Mongolia
Morocco
Netherlands
Norway

Pakistan
Poland
Portugal [incl. Azores, Madeira]
Romania
Ciscaucasia, Russian Federation
Dagestan, Russian Federation
European part, Russian Federation
Western Siberia, Russian Federation
Spain [incl. Baleares, Canary Islands]
Sweden
Switzerland
Syria
Tajikistan
Tunisia
Turkey
Turkmenistan
Ukraine [incl. Crimea]
United Kingdom
Yugoslavia

Which parts of the plant are used medicinally?

All the aeriel (above-ground) parts of the plant are used. There are even recipes for preparations involving the roots, but the more definitive herbals and scientific trials do not utilize the roots, only the stems, leaves, flowers, and buds.

Are any parts of the plant poisonous? Can my pets chew on it?

Unless you keep cows, sheep, or goats as pets, and have a pasture full of the herb, pet safety is not an issue. (St. John's Wort *has* produced sensitivity to the sun in cattle grazing on large amounts of the plant.) Other mammals tested on the herb have not experienced poisonous effects. As for humans, only excessively high doses of synthesized hypericin have produced similar phototoxic effects, unless a person is allergic to the herb. So far, there have not been any documented cases of hospitalization or death in humans associated with St. John's Wort. A few cows and sheep have not been so lucky, but your dog or cat should be fine if it dines on your supply.

When does the plant bloom?

Folklore holds that the flowers bloom on St. John the Baptist's birthday, which falls on June 24. Such precise timing is unlikely, but blooms will start to arrive on or very near that date. St. John's Wort seeds are harvested in early autumn; new plants are propagated from runners at this time, too.

Are any parts of the herb used in so-called legitimate medicines?

If by that, you mean synthesized drugs, then no. In the United States, no product made from the St. John's Wort plant is classified as a medication or drug, just a nutritional supplement. In Germany, extracts made from the *whole* aeriel plant are considered legitimate medicines. However, none of the herb's individual constituents has been isolated into a concentrated medication anywhere as yet. Until researchers locate the precise agents in the herb which work on depression (or other conditions), you won't see drugs made from any individual chemical parts of the plant.

How can it be possible that scientists don't know for sure how this herb works?

Actually scientists have a hard time with many herbs, not just St. John's Wort. It has proven difficult to find out which agents in an herb precipitate its healing actions, or whether it is some combination of two or more chemicals that provides an herb's medicinal properties. Researchers are learning more every day; sometimes the constituent originally thought to be the main player in an herb is upstaged at a later date by another with different actions. That may be the case with St. John's Wort as well, since recent studies have shown promise that xanthones may play a part in the herb's antidepressant actions, as well as hypericin. However, it's also important to keep in mind that the mechanism(s) of action of many widely used medications are not fully known, including mood-altering medications such as lithium and Prozac.

What's in a plant anyway? Does it have "ingredients"?

Well, yes, in fact plants do have "ingredients," which in scientific terms are called "constituents." Constituents are the basic chemicals which make up any living thing. The same constituent may be known by slightly different names; for example, citrol and citronellol are essentially the same thing. While this may sound confusing at first, it is actually organized that way to clarify precisely which species of plant harbors each chemical element. The variations in a name help clue scientists in that a chemical is derived from a particular plant. St. John's Wort has around 50 different chemicals in its makeup. It's a good idea to have some idea of the chemical constituents of plants like St. John's Wort, which are used medicinally, if only because so much of the literature about them tends to refer to these ingredients—often without the benefit of any explanation of what they are or the things they do (referred to as a chemical's "actions"). Also, some people may be aware of allergic reactions to certain chemicals, so having detailed information could prevent untoward reactions.

Basically, a plant is made up of a number of elements, some of which are found in our own human makeup: water is the primary ingredient in plants as well as people. We also share carbohydrates, fats, sugars, and mineral salts. Vitamins A and C are found in St. John's Wort. Alkaloids are also present and you can find complex proteins in plants like St. John's Wort. The fact that these constituents can be found in humans means that they not only play a role in the plant's survival, but also have a medicinal or nutritional effect in our bodies when we ingest the plants. As for constituents that may not sound so familiar, St. John's Wort contains active ingredients, such as hypericin, essential oils, flavonoids, and tannins. Resins and pectins are also part of the chemical mix. More information about some of these lesser-known constituents follows. Also, a number of the specific chemicals which make up those larger categories of constituents are listed in the following chart:

Basic Chemicals in St. John's Wort

Ascorbic Acid	Hyperoside	Phenol
Cadinene	Isoquercitrin	Phloroglucinol
Cadmium	Limonene	Pinene
Caryophyllene	Mannitol	Pseudohypericin
Chlorophyll	Myrcene	Pyrogallol
Choline	Myristic Acid	Quercetin
Epicatechin	N-Decanal	Quercitrin
Hyperforin	Palmitic Acid	Rutin
Hyperin	Pectin	Stearic Acid

*Source: USDA

What are the plant's active ingredients?

Pharmacologically active components of medicines, which are more commonly called "active ingredients," are those that produce some kind of healing or therapeutic effect. They are found in plants in combination with other, inactive materials. Components of St. John's Wort which are thought to be its active ingredients include:

- Dianthrones—These are pigments like hypericin, pseudohypericin, and their chemical cousins. They make up no more than .5% of extracts made from the plant, and often less, but may be the powerhouses behind the herb's antidepressant effects.
- Flavonoids—Enzymes which may perform several valuable actions in the body, flavonoids make up approximately 9% of the whole herb. Tannins are flavonoids, and they constitute about 10% of extracts from the herb, the highest proportion of the active ingredients.
- Volatile oils form about 1% of the total ingredients in a St. John's Wort extract.

What's a volatile oil? Is it the same as an essential oil?

Volatile oils are found in all aromatic plants, of which St. John's Wort is one. They are defined as oils that evaporate easily, and the concentration of these oils contributes to the plant's unique scent. Different levels of one oil or another may mean one plant of the same species has a different aroma from another even within the same family. St. John's Wort's essential oils are compounds of molecules called combination-terpenes and include humulene n-alkanes, methyl-2-octane, n-alkanols, alpha-pinene and other monoterpenes. If that is just so much jargon, consider that essential oils act as antifungals, preventing infections and bacteria growth in wounds. They also help stop buildup of mucus in the throat and lungs.

We use the term "essential oil" to refer to the product we get when volatile oils are removed from the plant through an extraction process, like soaking the herb in alcohol. Many perfumes use these essential oils, though I am not aware of any that utilize St. John's Wort. Concentrated oils from many aromatic plants are used in aromatherapy and are sold under the name essential oils. These should never be ingested, as they are so potent they can become toxic.

I keep hearing about flavonoids in St. John's Wort. What are they?

Flavonoids are sometimes referred to as flavanoids, flavones, and flavonols (although these may have slightly different chemical structures). Flavonoids are a group of semiessential polyphenolic compounds that, in St. John's Wort, include quercetin and the similarly named quercitin and quercitrin, rutin, hespiridin, kaempferol, and luteolin. Polyphenols are chemicals that affect the scent and taste of plants. Some flavonoids are pigments, the coloring agents in plants. Flavonoids are in every plant and tree, and over 4,000 varieties of flavonoids have so far been found in nature.

What do flavonoids do?

Flavonoids have similar roles in the St. John's Wort plant and in humans. They protect the plant from damage done by oxidation, a process that speeds decay. They also offer protection from fungi and bacteria. In humans, flavonoids likewise help stem the tide of oxidation, acting as an antioxidant (see more on this in Chapter Six—Beyond Depression). In addition, they have anti-inflammatory effects and may fight viruses by boosting the immune system. They can relax muscles in walls of blood vessels, which can improve the flow of blood in the cardiovascular system and prevent muscle spasms.

Bioflavonoids, a subcategory of flavonoids, help the body absorb vitamin C. Rutin is one such bioflavonoid, which also may help to repair weakened blood vessels. Initial studies indicate flavonoids may have some cancer-fighting effects, both through their actions against oxidation and also by inhibiting the production of the hormone estrogen, which could help prevent breast cancer. It appears that concentrations of flavonoids are highest in St. John's Wort plants found in northern locales, are most evident in the leaves, and most potent just before flowering when the plant is still in bud.

How is quercitin different from quercetin or quercitrin? Or are they the same thing? This is very confusing!

No wonder. The three are actually slightly different types of flavonoids. Like all flavonoids, they share some antioxidant effects. Named for a medieval scientist, quercetin is the most ubiquitous of the flavonoids; it's found in plants as in compounds that also contain sugars. Quercetin may be a free-radical scavenger and performs a variety of functions about which there is some controversy. For instance, it may have anti-inflammatory, antibacterial, antiviral, and antiallergenic properties, among others.

However, most of the current discussion in terms of quercetin in St. John's Wort is in the realm of its alleged antimutagenic action. That would mean it could slow the mutation of cells in an organism—mutations lead to a range of diseases, cancer among them. The controversy stems, for a large part, from the negative results of tests on mice and hamsters. So far tests of quercetin on rodents have failed to show mutagenic effects. Whether or not these tests can accurately mimic effects on humans is still debated, but currently, there is no scientific evidence that quercetin can prevent or treat cancer.

In contrast, quercitin does not have its cousin's anti-inflammatory effects, but instead is thought to promote higher levels of the "good" form of cholesterol known as HDL. And, finally, quercitrin has a different combination of actions—it is believed to possess sedative and, possibly, tumor-inhibiting effects. Again, these more dramatic alleged effects have not been proven.

I've heard about something called "procyanidins." How do they relate to flavonoids?

Procyanidins, also referred to as proanthocyanidins, are yet another subdivision of bioflavonoids that include the compounds catechin and epicatechin. These are also considered tannins because they have astringent properties. Astringents are chemicals that cause tissues to bind, dry, or "pucker." The various procyanidins appear to be highly effective antioxidants and may assist vitamin E in performing this function.

What actions do catechin and epicatechin have in St. John's Wort?

Catechin appears to be very active in bodily functions involving blood and the liver. Namely, it may help to inhibit blood clotting and strengthen capillary walls. Catechin is also an antioxidant. Epicatechin has many properties associated with it, among them: anti-inflammatory, antiviral, and antibacterial. Epicatechin also has been suggested to have antimutagenic effects.

What effect do tannins have?

The tannins in St. John's Wort include the flavonoids hyperoside, quercitin, rutin, and catechin. The name "tannin" originated because these chemicals are involved in the process of tanning hides—they affect the change in color of skin over time. There are many kinds of tannins, which are categorized as phenolic compounds. They produce the astringent effects of plants like St. John's Wort, which probably helps in the healing of wounds. The chemical also lays down a layer on the skin or mucus membranes, in essence sealing it off from bacteria and thus protecting it from infection. It also has anti-inflammatory actions. Cuts, rashes, and burns may thus be helped by tannins. In the digestive system, tannins in St. John's Wort may help reduce diarrhea. While some may have beneficial medicinal effects, other tannins are known to be toxic. They affect the production of some proteins and enzymes the body finds difficult to absorb.

I know rutin is a flavonoid found in St. John's Wort. Does it do anything special?

Rutin is a flavonoid routinely found in more complex plants. Like the other flavonoids, it has some antioxidant qualities, as well as the potential for strengthening capillaries, which are the tiniest and most fragile blood vessels. It's this action that has led to St. John's Wort's anecdotal application for varicose veins, among other things.

Is hyperforin the same thing as hypericin?

Actually, hyperforin is a phloroglucinol derivative, not a dianthrone pigment like hypericin. Uh-huh, right, you're probably thinking. More to the point, the chemical hyperforin does not have the antidepressant properties of hypericin, but rather is thought to be a potent germ fighter. It may play a part in making St. John's Wort effective in healing wounds and also in the herb's sedative effects.

I've heard something about xanthones being the ingredient that works on depression. Is that what they do in St. John's Wort?

For a long time, hypericin was thought to be the lone monoamine oxidase inhibitor (MAOI) in St. John's Wort (MAOIs help raise levels of serotonin in the body, enhancing feelings of happiness or pleasure). But more recent tests have shown that might not be the case, as xanthones might have similar serotonin-boosting properties. In fact, hypericin does not seem to act as an MAOI when isolated from other ingredients in the herb. More testing is needed to determine the specific role of xanthones in depression therapy, both alone and in combination with hypericin. Xanthones may have other functions as well: treating diarrhea; helping to lessen water-retention; and a virus- and bacteria-fighting agent.

What exactly is hypericin? I hear it's the ingredient that works on depression.

Hypericin is described in a number of ways chemically: as a dianthone or dianthrone derivative, anthroquinone, aromatic polycyclic dione, or a napthodianthrone. These are terms based on chemical structure that to the nonchemist have little meaning. More simply, hypericin is a photodynamic red pigment, which means it is a chemical that gets more potent when exposed to light and that it helps give the herb its bright, insect-attracting color. As a pigment, it also makes the plant useful in the production of dyes for silk and wool.

But more importantly, hypericin could be considered the herb's "marker" agent in depression therapy, because it's likely hypericin is one of the chief chemicals responsible for the herb's antidepressant effects. When calculating the 0.3% of hypericin found in the commercial preparations of the herb, scientists are including not just hypericin itself, but close chemical relatives which have many of the same properties, such as pseudohypericin, protohypericin, cyclopseudohypericin, emodinathranol, and hyperico-dehydro-dianthrol. One of those or, possibly, some combination of them may be behind the monoamine oxidase inhibition effects of St. John's Wort which lead to higher levels of serotonin, since recent tests have indicated that hypericin alone does not act as a powerful inhibitor.

Hypericin, then, must work on depression in a more subtle way than simple MAO inhibition, or only in combination with other St. John's Wort constituents. Even when the other diathrones are not counted, there is some disagreement over how much hypericin is found in the herb; sources rate levels as anything from as little as .00095% to as much as .5% of the total content of the herb's leaves, with flowers averaging .24% of hypericin in their components.

One reason for the controversy may be the simple fact that crops of the herb collected in different locations always vary in levels of active ingredients, owing to environmental factors. The other dianthrones, like pseudohypericin, isohypericin, and protohypericin, may be antivirals. Their structures may look alike, but there are some essential differences in the way they work pharmaceutically. For instance, it's not clear whether pseudohypericin has any effect on depression, although it may be involved in whatever impact St. John's Wort has on the immune system.

Hypericin and the other dianthrones may play a role in other functions besides depression therapy. Hypericin is classed as an anthroquinone, chemicals known to affect the wavelike contractions of the muscle in the bowel walls, which push wastes through the intestines. So anthroquinones like hypericin may account for the reports that St. John's Wort aids in digestion.

Do the herb's resins and pectins have any medicinal effects?

Pectins play a role in the smooth running of your digestive system, as they are substances that add bulk to the diet, like dietary fiber, which helps the work of the bowels. They may assist in digestion by helping to stimulate the production of insulin. Resins are plant oils that operate in the plant as a balm that fills damaged plant tissues and prevents water loss. Resins also make plants taste unappealing to grazing predators. Medicinally, resins may serve a variety of functions. Some resins help aid in the healing of wounds, protecting the skin from bacteria and harmful microorganisms. Other resins act as aromatic expectorants, diuretics, or antioxidants. Not much testing has been done to indicate if any of these functions are served by the pectins and resins in St. John's Wort, but certainly the therapeutic properties described have been attributed to the herb.

What is a glycoside?

Glycosides are a form of complex sugar. For instance, when a flavononid bonds with a sugar it becomes a flavonoid glycoside. Several of St. John's Wort's basic constituents form these glycoside compounds. Glycosides help ensure a plant's survival by producing valuable compounds that help plants withstand attacks from the animals that might eat them. In humans, glycosides affect cardiac functions and are sometimes used in the treatment of arrhythmia, disorders of cardiac rhythm and tachycardia, as well as hypotension. Certain glycosides are also used in asthma therapies. Some of the glycosides found in St. John's Wort are the flavones and flavonols (or quercetin glycosides) such as kaempferol, luteolin, quercetin, quercitrin, and rutin. Lesser-known glycosides in the herb include cyanogenic glycosides, glycosinolates, coumarins, cardiac glycosides, saponins, isoflavones and coumestans (phytoestrogens), nitroglycosides, and vicine/convicine.

I notice St. John's Wort has vitamins A and C. What do those two vitamins do?

Vitamin C is present, in some degree, in all plants. This is a good thing, since our only source of this vitamin is food—the human body doesn't manufacture vitamin C. Yet we need it as a source of ascorbic acid, to promote a number of functions, including the strengthening of skin, bones, teeth, and capillary walls. Vitamin C is also an active participant in the body's healing reaction to cuts, bruises, and other skin disruptions. You can see some of these effects in St. John's Wort. Vitamin C helps in the fight against oxidation as well, by stopping certain chemicals called nitrates (present in aged, canned, cured, or processed meats, some vegetables like beans, and air pollutants like tobacco smoke and smog) from forming into compounds that speed decay and promote cancers. Some of the bioflavonoids in St. John's Wort, like quercetin, rutin, and hespridin, help your body absorb vitamin C more efficiently.

Vitamin A is better known as beta-carotene, a nutrient that, like St. John's Wort, has had a lot of press recently. Commonly associated with orange and green vegetables, vitamin A is also found in other plants, including herbs. Recent hoopla has centered around the possibility that beta-carotene may help prevent certain lung and oral cancers. But several more well established effects of the vitamin have been noted, including improved night vision; healthier skin, bones, and teeth; stimulation of white blood cell production; and stronger defenses against infections of the nose, mouth, throat, and lungs.

I've heard St. John's Wort is photodynamic. What does that mean?

It means that certain of the plant's basic components, hypericin for example, perform some therapeutic actions better when it has been exposed to light. That may mean that plants grown in sunnier conditions have more potent levels of hypericin; it's still not confirmed. What has been proven is that some animals become far more sensitive to sunlight after eating large amounts of the herb. This seems the case only in cattle, however, since rodents and other mammals have not demonstrated this effect. Similar reactions have not been documented in humans using the natural herb taken orally in standard amounts. However, photosensitivity has been observed in studies using synthesized extracts of hypericin administered intravenously in very large doses.

I saw reports that St. John's Wort can be used on depression, but my mom uses it on cuts. Plus I've heard it works on cold symptoms. What else does it do?

If you're going by word-of-mouth accounts, St. John's Wort has all three of the therapeutic effects mentioned—antidepressant, anti-inflammatory, and expectorant. But that's just the tip of the iceberg if you go by tales passed down through generations and preserved in herbals. In fact, anecdotal accounts credit St. John's Wort with an extraordinarily broad range of therapeutic effects, benefiting people with conditions as diverse (alphabetically) as allergies to zerostomia (dry mouth). In addition, St. John's Wort is used in an alcohol-based bluish red dye for silks, an alum-based beige dye for wool, and a slightly bitter addition to salad greens.

But be warned! (My intention here is not to promote a modern version of "snake oil.") There is nothing but anecdotal information to support many of these claims—stories casually passed from one person to another, not reports that have been systematically and scientifically documented. Even anecdotal evidence is slight in many cases. Still, the whole parade of "cures" gets trotted out at one point or another by organizations selling the herb and well-intentioned enthusiasts who wish to promote natural remedies or alternative approaches to medicine. In fact, the only indications I have seen for some of these uses have been in lists in older herbals or ads. (You'll find more detailed information about the use of St. John's Wort and many of these conditions in Chapter Six—Beyond Depression.) But first, we'll take a look at the use which is getting most of the attention these days: depression therapy.

TWO

◆

"The Blues," Major Depression, and Other Forms of Mild to Moderate Depression

Whenever a "new" remedy like St. John's Wort comes along, I look at it as an opportunity. For an all-too-brief period, the remedy focuses attention on how common depression is and just how debilitating its effects are. People struggling with depression, those who have depressed friends, relatives, and coworkers, and those who help treat it, seize on the intense interest generated by a new therapy as a chance to inform and educate others about the disorder it treats. While the main focus and all the attendant hoopla will obviously be on the herb, some light will be thrown on depression itself. At the least, all the notice may get people talking about the disorder and this will help to reduce the stigma. Sufferers who ordinarily never discuss their condition, might begin tentatively to ask others about the herb—and be surprised to find out coworkers, family members, or friends use it in their own battles with depression.

They shouldn't be surprised. It's ironic that a sense of crippling isolation and loneliness, an emotion often associated with depression, should be a hallmark of this most common of illnesses. As a sufferer, you may feel like you are alone in your pain, but the reality is that at least 10 to 15 percent of all adults report suffering an episode of depression at one time or another. Mind you, this is not the blues or "normal" sadness we are talking about, this is a bona fide clinical episode of major depression! Over *17 million* people each year in the U.S. alone will experience some form of depressive illness. So you are far from being alone. In this country, depression's symptoms are the number one reason people visit their family physicians. The disorder's ripple effect has an impact on the lives of millions more, as family members, friends, and co-workers all suffer some of the consequences of the illness's disabling effects. These effects are most apparent among the partners, spouses, and children of depressed people, who may be on the receiving end of anger attacks, violent behavior, neglect, or, most commonly, emotional withdrawal.

Yet many people still will not admit to the possibility of having this serious illness nor will they discuss it with their closest family and friends, let alone seek treatment. In fact, it's estimated that at any given time only about a third of those suffering are getting professional treatment for depression, choosing instead to keep quiet about their condition, attempting to treat themselves, or seeking medical help for less specific symptom complaints (e.g., "stress," insomnia, or chronic fatigue). That's a frustrating statistic, since research has shown that 80-90% of those who do seek professional help for depression can be successfully treated. I am particularly concerned about the possibility that St. John's Wort's over-the-counter availability will, inadvertently, increase the tendency for depressed people not to seek professional help. Even the most powerful "mainstream" treatments do not help more than 70 to 80 percent of those who receive a good trial of therapy, and the best chances of success come when treatment is preceded by a careful diagnostic interview, a review of general health status, and, if deemed necessary, a complete medical history, physical exam, and appropriate laboratory studies. So, at this stage of the game, there is reason to worry that self-treatment with St. John's Wort will override more definitive therapy.

It's a safe bet that even if St. John's Wort is all it's cracked up to be, the herbal remedy won't help more than 50 to 60 percent of depressed people, which is the typical response rate for depressed outpatients treated with standard antidepressants. There are clearly limits to what the herbal remedy can do, especially with the more severe forms of depression. Long-term studies also may show up some as of yet unrecognized flaw in treatment with the herb that could prove the whole thing to be a boondoggle.

Hopefully, though, interest in finding something to help relieve their pain will motivate people to find out more about what's causing the crippling symptoms in the first place. However, I *do not* believe that anyone should use a remedy unless he or she is first diagnosed and then comes to understand the condition it is supposed to treat.

So, let's talk about depression.

The first thing you should know is that depression is what's known as a biopsychosocial disorder. It is an illness that affects the mind, brain, body, and spirit, or soul. Depression may have chemical, psychological, and environmental causes—and affects not just your emotional responses but your physical well-being, through its actions on sleep, appetite, immune system, and other body functions. These are the reasons behind the disorder's wide-ranging symptoms and why depression is linked to many other conditions and diseases.

When people speak of depression as a condition, not just a feeling state, they are most often talking about clinical syndromes technically labeled major depressive disorder, or dysthymic disorder. However, the syndrome of depression also can be caused by general medical diseases, like hypothyroidism or a brain tumor, or by a wide range of commonly prescribed medications, including some blood pressure drugs, birth control pills, and steroid hormones. A syndrome of depression also commonly follows a prolonged period of alcohol or drug abuse.

A syndrome is a group of signs, symptoms, and characteristics that ''hang together'' in a meaningful way. For example, coughing, fever, and difficulty breathing help define the syndrome of pneumonia. In turn, a medical syndrome may have many causes (e.g., pneumonia could be caused by a virus, a particular bacterium or fungus, or by aspirating liquid into your lungs). Syndromes that have more specific known causes are commonly referred to as diseases, whereas more biopsychosocial illnesses like depression are referred to as disorders.

The key concept implied in a ''clinical depression'' is that the disorder warrants professional (i.e., in the clinic) treatment. Frankly, I think we use the expression ''clinical'' to help convey that the disorder should be taken seriously, i.e., not simply a case of feeling "down in the dumps."

In addition to major depression and dysthymia, the other types include an aspect called *bipolar disorder* (also called manic-depressive disorder). Major depression and dysthymia are the most prevalent, together accounting for about 80 to 90 percent of all people diagnosed with primary depressive disorders. However, I'm aware of patients in all the categories of mood disturbances who are attempting to treat themselves with St. John's Wort, with widely varying levels of success.

Most of these depressive disorders, about which people commonly have questions, will be addressed briefly in this chapter. You'll find some answers here, but to get a complete picture of how depression or other forms of mental illnesses relate to your specific situation, talk to your doctor. You are unique, and your expression of any given illness will be just as individual. Find out more about what's got you in its grip. Knowledge is the first step to regain control over your health and emotional well-being.

My husband isn't trying to be cruel but he asks me why I just can't seem to cope. How can I explain it to him—and to myself?

It's not easy explaining depression to someone who is not experiencing a daily struggle with its symptoms and impairments. Sadness is a normal emotional response to loss, and we are programmed to recognize the facial expressions of sadness and respond supportively. This is essential to human survival—imagine, if you will, trying not to respond to a crying child who is lost and alone. Basically, everyone knows what sadness feels like; some people believe that they "know" the natural remedies to sadness—distracting oneself, seeking the support of others, or doing something to solve the problem. Your spouse, for example, might say, "When I get depressed, I just pick myself up by my bootstraps and get moving." If only it were that easy! It is very likely that your spouse is confusing normal sadness with depression. To try to give others some sense of how coping has been taken out of a depressed person's control, I sometimes use the metaphor of a car speeding toward a brick wall: If you are going too fast, it doesn't matter how great your brakes are—you are still going to hit the wall. Likewise, if you are only cruising at 30 miles an hour but have defective brakes, you'll still hit that wall.

That's what it's like for people with depression. For some people, even smaller, seemingly manageable stresses become amplified by the illness—just as stepping on the gas will amplify the speed of a car to the point of danger. So no matter how good these people's coping mechanisms usually are, it won't help. Inevitably, they're going to react to the stress with an equally amplified response—a bad crash. For other people, the stress response itself isn't amplified; instead, the brain's way of dampening normal stress responses is somehow impaired—their brakes simply aren't functioning. With depression, it may be a question of either of these malfunctions—brakes or gas—but about one thing there is no question, sooner or later sufferers *will* hit a brick wall and crash.

Another consequence of a prolonged and exaggerated stress response is a decrease in the capacity to enjoy things, the energy to do things, and the ability to plan and execute solutions to complex problems. Thus, when the depressed person tries to cope, they find that their efforts are ineffective. This adds to their sense of feeling out of control, weak, and a failure.

These small steps toward understanding are important from a treatment standpoint. For people usually begin just as you have, with the notion that if they can only "get it together," they can solve their problems. Just cope, they tell themselves. But, of course, if they truly have a clinical depressive disorder, that hasn't worked. There is something in their biochemical and psychological makeup that prevents that from happening. So the next step is to get professional help—basically employ someone to help get them in gear and to assist in solving those problems.

Ask your husband and yourself: Why is acknowledging that something inside you is malfunctioning perceived as an admission of weakness? You and your husband would get help if your car were having trouble with its engine or brakes— you'd do it even more quickly if you knew there was a brick wall at the end of your street. If you couldn't fix your car's brakes yourself, why would you assume you could fix something as complex as how your brain is functioning on your own?

What's the difference between depression and just plain feeling blue?

Most of us have experienced "the blues" at some point in our lives: when our parents die, when a lover walks out on us, or we get unfairly fired or professionally embarrassed or humiliated. We don't call that a disorder because being confronted with a bad situation that hasn't got any kind of immediate resolution is, unfortunately, a common part of the human experience. If it's death, we call it grief, if it's a setback in love or work, we call it a bad time. Typically, time heals the wound and we feel better soon. When we have good support, it usually doesn't knock us out of our life's trajectory.

When compared to a major depressive episode, the blues are less intense, have fewer associated symptoms, cause little or no impairment in the tasks of everyday life, and last a much shorter time.

If you did approach a doctor during such a troubled time and she determined that you had no tendency toward depression, that the period of dejection showed signs of being temporary and your symptoms could be tracked back to a very specific event, your condition might be labeled an "adjustment disorder" or a "reactive" mood disturbance—"the blues" in laymen's terms. If you were experiencing grief, and it caused you to miss work and sleep, but other symptoms of depression were not present, it might be labeled "complicated grief." In either case, your symptoms would be easily treatable and you and your doctor could be reasonably confident that the emotional pain would pass.

Even though one person's expression of grief or adjustment to a stressful event may be very different from another's— tears, anger, stoicism, indifference, a constant craving for "comfort" foods high in sugar and starch—still, these are normal, appropriate responses. A healthy person experiencing these symptoms as a result of some traumatic life event can continue performing everyday functions and is not incapacitated. It is only when responses to an event are extreme to the point of disabling the sufferer, when symptoms persist every day for more than two weeks or get worse, and eventually prevent that person from engaging in normal day-to-day activities, that the condition has reached a new level, that of an episode of major depression. Its disabling impact is one of the things that distinguishes clinical depression from a simple case of the blues.

Keep in mind that someone currently in an episode of depression has most likely had similar periods of depression in the past that ebbed and flowed, even if symptoms had never before reached the present level of intensity. There might be something about this particular time in a person's life, though—symptoms feel worse or are taking a greater toll on the person's day-to-day functioning, or maybe the strategies that used to work don't any longer—that crosses the line between the blues and depression.

I've been feeling incredibly low ever since a death in the family. How do I know it's not depression?

You are not alone in being confused. When well-meaning people insist that you'll feel better "soon," but you are still tearful or numb weeks later, you should become concerned. It's all a question of time and severity. Many people experiencing grief feel a profound sorrow that does not disperse after weeks or more. Noticeable weight loss and nights of insomnia also are common expressions of bereavement.

Our love relationships are an essential part of the human experience and when one of these attachments is broken, the emotional impact can be devastating. When you first receive the blow of a loved one's death, it may seem as if the sadness will never go away, that you will never feel better. But does the profound sadness seem to soften a little as the days pass? Are you eventually able to eat and rest? Can you go about the basic business of life without a significant loss of function? Can you experience pleasure, show a sense of humor, or distract yourself from your misery? The truth is that most people do feel better within a few weeks, without any more involved therapy than the simple passage of time and comfort from loved ones and friends. Symptomatic treatment to relieve anxiety or insomnia also can help.

Although grief is the most common or universal emotional response that can serve as a model of depression, other losses and insults can have similar effects on our well being. In addition to our basic needs for attachments and support, to have good self-esteem most people also need to have a sense of competence or worth about their abilities to contribute to their family or society—not unrealistic expectations, mind you, nor a slavish devotion to performance at the expense of attachments to others. Thus, a pattern of underachievement or a dramatic or humiliating failure at school or in the workplace can be as stressful as the death of a loved one. Often, it is the sense that the problem is unsolvable, perhaps coupled with the belief that the problem will have far-reaching and lasting implications that catapult a normal response to a setback to a more extreme disturbance that warrants professional treatment.

But if the feelings connected to your distress are not going away, you may have passed seamlessly into an episode of major depression, and you may need more help than time and support can provide. An episode of major depression might be diagnosed if profound emotional reactions continue for more than two weeks at the same intensity or if you cannot return to everyday activities after the first shock of the death. Typically, there is also a significant loss of self-esteem and other symptoms of depression. Not surprisingly, though, the distinction between grief and depression is sometimes difficult to make, especially since every person's method of dealing with bereavement is different and can, in fact, vary widely from culture to culture. The herb's role in the more complex biopsychological response of true depression is not yet fully defined, and may depend on the severity scale of the episode.

I feel like I have depression. But how can I be *sure*?

You might not be able to and you shouldn't even try to make this diagnosis on your own. If you're at all unsure about your mental health, you should be talking to a physician or therapist.

Are there easy-to-identify symptoms of a depressive disorder?

Look at any listing of the warning signs of mental illness and you'll see that there are some classic symptoms, including the emotional symptom referred to as a depressed mood. But these symptoms only become definitive identifiers of a specific condition when put into a context—when someone knowledgeable about psychiatric disorders looks at them in the bigger picture of your life and overall physical health. That's why depression is not a condition you should attempt to self-diagnose. The symptoms are too easily misread and misunderstood. They could, in fact, be caused by a number of other conditions or diseases. Only a doctor who knows your medical and psychiatric history, and has eliminated all other possible organic causes, should make a diagnosis.

When your doctor makes a diagnosis of depression, you can then rate the severity of your depression using the following charts. One approach is to tally your symptoms and the severity of each symptom.

COULD YOU BE IN A MAJOR DEPRESSION EPISODE?

I have felt this way or experienced these symptoms *most every day* for at least two consecutive weeks (check the appropriate box for each question):

	YES	MAYBE	NO	SYMPTOM LIST
1.	❑	❑	❑	I feel sad, down, empty, blue, or tearful.
2.	❑	❑	❑	I am not interested in things or experience little pleasure in all or almost all of my activities.
3.	❑	❑	❑	I have either a decreased or an increased appetite.
or	❑	❑	❑	My weight has changed by 5 percent or more in the past month without trying to diet or "bulk up."
4.	❑	❑	❑	I either have insomnia or sleep too much.
5.	❑	❑	❑	I have been so slowed down or agitated that others have noticed the change.
6.	❑	❑	❑	I am really tired. Fatigue has become a problem.
7.	❑	❑	❑	I have thoughts about being worthless *or* about my mistakes and shortcomings.
8.	❑	❑	❑	My concentration is decreased *or* it's hard to think clearly or make decisions.
9.	❑	❑	❑	I have recurrent thoughts about death or I am thinking about suicide.

	YES	MAYBE	NO	SYMPTOM LIST
10.	❑	❑	❑	One or more of the above symptoms are causing me to have problems at home, at work or school, or in some other area.
11.	❑	❑	❑	As far as I know, these symptoms are caused by another medical illness or condition.
12.	❑	❑	❑	I do feel this way as a result of recent or current use of alcohol or some other drug of abuse.

[*Source: *Diagnostic and Statistical Manual of Mental Disorders, Fourth Edition (DSM IV)*, American Psychiatric Association, 1994.

This checklist is not meant to replace a clinical interview by a trained mental health professional. People who have a diagnosis of major depressive disorder answer "yes" to either question 1 or 2, and "yes" to at least five of the first nine questions. If so, you also have to answer "yes" to question 10. If you think that your symptoms are caused by another medical problem or medication (question 11) or drug or alcohol use (question 12), you may still have a depressive syndrome that would benefit from treatment, even though you might not technically qualify for the diagnosis of major depressive syndrome.

The clinical syndromes of depression are categorized as mood or affective disorders because the defining characteristics center around extreme, exaggerated, and/or distorted expressions of normal emotions or moods. Unlike normal sadness or unhappiness, however, the mood change in depression is more persistent (most of the day, most every day) and has broader effects. Also, unlike normal sadness, the syndrome is further defined by similarly persistent disturbances of energy, sleep, appetite, interest or enthusiasm, concentration, and body movements (usually slowing, but sometimes agitation). There are many different expressions or variations of these signs and symptoms, which probably affect both our diversity as human beings and the multiple causes of depression.

Several common variations of clinical depression are listed and described on the following pages. Most importantly, St. John's Wort has not been studied in the more severe forms of major depressive disorder, including melancholia and psychotic depression. St. John's Wort also has not been studied as a preventative, long-term treatment for recurrent depression, nor has it been studied systematically in manic depression (also known as bipolar affective disorder). The most common forms of clinical depression are major depressive disorder and dysthymia. The course or ebb and flow of these conditions are illustrated in the accompanying figures. Notice that for manic depression, the time chart has two "poles"—one for mania and the other for depression.

CLINICAL SUBTYPES AND
PRESENTATIONS OF DEPRESSION

Dysthymia: a syndrome defined by two years of unremitting symptoms that are not severe and/or persistent enough to be declared a major depressive disorder (MDD).

Recurrent ("Unipolar") Major Depression: a syndrome defined by at least two lifetime episodes of major depression.

"Double" Depression: dysthymia that is complicated by one or more major depressive episodes.

Melancholia: a more severe episode of depression with prominent insomnia, weight loss, loss of pleasure, and disturbances of movement (slowing or agitation). More common past age fifty, melancholia is also known as biological, "vital," endogenous, and autonomous depression.

Bipolar (Manic) Depression: periods of mania that have been preceded or followed by a major depressive episode.

Atypical Features: a milder and often early onset disorder, these depressive episodes are defined by "reverse" symptoms such as overeating and sleeping, weight gain.

Seasonal Pattern: a regular pattern of episodes of mood disorders, usually characterized by depressive episodes in the fall and winter and mania (or its milder form, hypomania) in the spring or summer.

Now, remember: don't look at any list of depression symptoms and suddenly decide, "I've got that *and* that—I must be mentally ill!" Charts and lists are not provided for self-diagnosis, only as red flags warning you it may be time to see a doctor. A qualified physician can help you to determine if

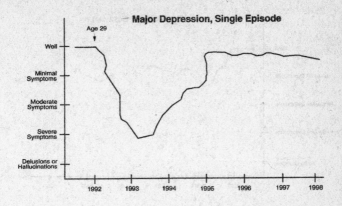

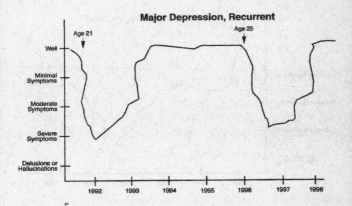

there are physical causes for any of these symptoms. Moreover, when it comes to diagnosis, things become complicated by the simple fact that other factors are also at play, any or all of which could confound an easy identification: Age, sex, menstrual phases, nutritional habits, and environmental elements like the time of day or season might influence a person's symptoms. Even a knowledgeable herbalist or homeopath might not be well-trained in distinguishing a definite symptom from a perfectly normal variation in response to stress. Let someone with a background in the study of psychiatric or psy-

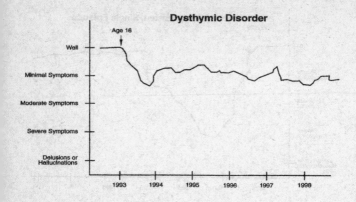

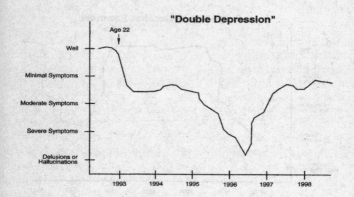

chological disorders help you determine the interplay of all the differing factors involved in a diagnosis of depression.

So is depression chemical or mental? What causes it?

It is actually impossible to separate the two. *All* of your body responses can be thought of as chemical—breathing is chemical, reaching to turn a page involves a complicated interconnected series of electrochemical connections between the brain and the nerves and muscles involved in the task.

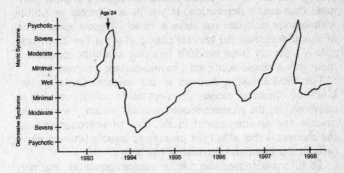

Bipolar Affective Disorder

Today, we call reactions involving nerve cells, or neurons, neurochemical. So, thinking is neurochemical and emotions are neurochemical. Any function performed by the brain involves neurochemical processes. So if someone says your depression is all in your mind, you might agree with the words if not the meaning.

Over the centuries, the distinction between the physical, the chemical, or the mental has provided a useful way of understanding or explaining our being. This convenience is now obsolete, even though we hold on to its beautiful simplicity tenaciously. For example, the study of the brain and its neurochemical messengers is grouped within "biological psychiatry," even though thoughts, feelings, and memories are also biological processes. In any event, biological psychiatry would also include studies of inherited or genetic influences, the actions of various medications, electroconvulsive therapy, and changes in hormones and sleep physiology associated with depression.

We do know that there must be some sort of genetic connection to depression, because a tendency toward the disorder appears to be hereditary. Heredity, not just common upbringing, can be inferred from studies comparing identical and fraternal (nonidentical) twins and the risks faced by those "adopted-away" from their biological parents. It is not yet known what chemical process in genetic DNA is involved, and it seems likely that what is inherited is a tendency, or vulnerability, not the illness itself. Manic depression is more heritable than major depression; if you have a parent or sibling with bipolar disorder you have a 10 to 20 times greater risk of this illness than the general public. But a 10 to 20 percent risk is a far cry from the 50% risk that would be expected *if* there was a single dominant "manic-depression gene."

The most credible theories at the moment focus on two kinds of chemical causes for depression, often working in combination: the aforementioned genetic tendency toward the disease and an impairment in the flow of neurotransmitters, the chemicals that affect the passage of signals between nerve cells in the brain and the rest of the body.

To fully understand the role of neurotransmitters, you may need a Ph.D. in basic brain and central nervous system (CNS) biology and several lifetimes of research and scholarship. But, for the rest of us, here's the Cliff's Notes version of the way it works: The central nervous system is made up of nerve cells which carry messages from the peripheral and autonomic nerves in organs and tissues up through the spinal cord to the brain, and vice versa. These bundles, or tracts, of nerves carry every kind of sensory input received by the body to the brain. Aside from very simple neuron reflexes, it is the brain's job to "process" and interpret sensory data. Interpretation includes basic perception ("This is hot." "That is too loud.") and the possible meanings associated with those perceptions ("It was rude to make that loud noise."). There are also motor areas of the brain that initiate and control our voluntary movements. Like insects or lizards, we tend to move towards things that give us pleasure or sate our desires, and away from things that give us pain. We mammals are distinguished by our live-born young, warm-blooded circulation, body hair, and nursing mothers and, as primates, by our very long time to physical maturity and giant cerebral cortex. And, we humans differ from the remainder of the primates by the size and complexity of our brains, as exemplified by the use of formal and abstract thought and spoken and written language. But, we're getting ahead of ourselves.

Neurons are separated by tiny spaces called synapses, so in order for a message to pass from one cell to another, neurotransmitters are released to "jump" the gap. Once released by the cell sending the message, the neurotransmitter may connect to a receptor on the cell receiving the signal. The common metaphor used to describe this action is that of a key and lock, neurotransmitters acting the role of the keys and receptor sites in the nerve cells being the locks. One of the reasons the key analogy is used is because neurotransmitters are chemically matched to specific receptor sites, sort of like a key is to its lock. So, when a message is being sent, neurotransmitters flood the synapse, slotting into their matching receptor sites. The message then may ride this connection from one nerve cell to the next, or it may trigger changes within the cell itself. Different types of neurotransmitters pass along different types of messages.

Once neurotransmitters are received by receptor cells, they may be processed or "cleaned up" by enzymes, or they may be reabsorbed back into the sending cell, a process called reuptake. By stopping or slowing the reuptake action—or by inhibiting the cleanup process—medications can alter the signaling process. Basically, these types of effects may amplify or strengthen a weak signal. Hence the term "reuptake inhibitor," or monoamine oxidase inhibitor, which you'll so often run across in discussions on depression.

There are different kinds of neurotransmitters. So far, serotonin, norepinephrine, and dopamine appear to be those which play the biggest role in depression. Acetylcholine may also be involved.

Acetylcholine is a small neurotransmitter used by nerve cells that carry messages relating to motor and glandular functions. In experimental studies, high levels of acetylcholine can mimic some of the changes in sleep and appetite associated with depression. More importantly, many common antidepressant side effects are caused by inhibiting acetylcholine effects ("anticholinergic"), which is not necessary to treat depression.

Serotonin is also a chemical mediator. This means that in addition to its regular functions, serotonin has an effect on other chemicals in your body, most notably the *endorphins*. Commonly called "nature's painkillers," endorphins modify messages of pain-perception, pleasure, and emotional well-being. You can imagine their importance in depression. When serotonin levels are low, endorphins do not appear to function as effectively.

Nerve cells in the brain that use serotonin are involved in regulating sleep, appetite, libido, body temperature, and hormone release. Generally, serotonin neurons have inhibitory effects that keep us balanced and protect us from getting overstimulated.

There is much evidence that chronic stress can reduce brain serotonin levels *and* that people with low serotonin levels have problems with impulsivity and moodiness. Serotonin levels fall when a primate loses social dominance, and rise again when he is "promoted." Many medications for depressions block reuptake of serotonin or inhibit the enzymes that break it down.

Norepinephrine is a hormone released by the adrenal medullary glands. It controls blood flow by contracting vessels, thus increasing blood pressure. But norepinephrine also has an effect on messages of pleasure and pain. In the brain, norepinephrine tracts are involved in "awakeness" or arousal and bursts of norepinephrine cell activity will trigger the famous "fight or flight" response. Prolonged stress also will deplete brain norepinephrine levels. Furthermore, stress stimulates the production of more hormones, the most famous of which is cortisol. Cortisol is released from the adrenal cortex and exerts anti-inflammatory and stabilizing effects. Although a high cortisol level is good during times of temporary stress, it can cause problems if sustained for too long. Some studies suggest that elevated cortisol levels may be "shut down" or corrected by more powerful treatments (like electroconvulsive therapy or some forms of pharamacotherapy). It appears that people with prolonged elevations of cortisol also are less likely to respond to placebo or psychotherapy.

Adding to the complexity are a number of other chemical connections. Dopamine is the neurochemical that is primarily involved in the brain's reward or pleasure center (along with norepinephrine) and it is involved in concentration, problem-solving, and speed of muscle movements. Dopamine is more often talked about in schizophrenia (too much dopamine stimulation can cause hallucinations).

Melatonin may be another chemical culprit in some forms of depression. It is a hormone produced by the pineal glands.

Melatonin has a significant role in maintaining the sleep-wake cycle and higher levels commonly precede sleep. Some people who sleep too much when depressed—especially those who have recurrent winter depressions—appear to have an abnormality in the daily melatonin rhythm.

Finally, we have to remember that there is an incredibly broad range of mood and anxiety disorders, and even the subcategory of major depressive disorder can span a pretty wide spectrum of severity. Most researchers believe that the psychobiological factors involved in major depression and bipolar disorder are different too. Alternate chemicals may be involved, as well as diverse nervous-system malfunctions. So far, biological abnormalities have been harder to spot in cases of milder major depression than they have been in cases that fall under the categories of bipolar, delusional, and melancholic mood disorders. Does that mean that major depression is all in your head? Probably not, but the type of chemical disturbances may be more subtle, and it may be more responsive to therapies that don't inhibit neurotransmitter reuptake or the enzyme monoamine oxidase.

It all seems complex, and it is. Even this brief synopsis of the chemical connection demonstrates why it has been so hard for scientists and doctors to pin the rap on any one, single chemical cause. It is highly unlikely that depression's incredibly diverse symptoms could all be traceable to one single biochemical abnormality. Still, virtually all the biological theories involve disturbances of the parts of the brain governing sleep, appetite, emotion, and the experience of pleasurable feelings. Take a look at the chart below, which summarizes these chemicals and their associates:

Neurotransmitters involved in depression	Other chemicals affected by these transmitters	Enzymes which break down the neurotransmitters	Some of the drugs that impact on these transmitters
Norepinephrine (NE)	Dopamine Dopa Tyrosine Phenylalanine	Monoaminexoidase (MAO) Catechol-O-methyl transferase (COMT)	Prazosine Clonidine Yohimbine Despiramine Nortriptyline

Neurotransmitters involved in depression	Other chemicals affected by these transmitters	Enzymes which break down the neurotransmitters	Some of the drugs that impact on these transmitters
Serotonin (5-HT or 5-hydroxytryptamine)	L-Tryptophan 5-Hydroxytryptophan (5-HTP)	MAO	Ipsapirone Ketanserin Ondansertone Fenfluramine SSRIs
Dopamine (DA)	Dopa Phenylalanine Tyrosine	MAO COMT DBH	Raclopride Apomorphine Quinpirol Clozaprine
Acetylcholine (ACh)	Choline Phosphatidylcholine	Cholinesterase	Atropine Belladonna Nicotine

I hear about serotonin all the time. Just how important is it in treating depression?

Every day we are learning more about the complex processes involving neurochemicals like serotonin. What we do know is that serotonin is released when the walls of blood cells are injured in some way. In addition to this damage-control reaction, serotonin is an important element in the regulation of sleeping and eating patterns and sexual behavior. It also helps control messages concerning digestion, muscle tissues, and the contraction of blood vessels. It is implicated in regulating body temperature, hormone release, and inhibiting aggressive impulses. Finally, serotonin has effects on other biochemicals like endorphins. Monoamine oxidase is the enzyme responsible for breaking down serotonin.

Which of these actions are involved in the complex tangle of mood disturbances? Are serotonin levels too low in people with depression? That's hard to say at the moment. We're still not completely sure which is responsible or if it's some combination of actions. Nor are scientists absolutely sure this whole process is really at the root of depression or just related in a secondary way. Just the same, there's a lot of evidence that serotonin is disturbed in many cases of depression and antidepressants that selectively enhance serotonin have definite therapeutic effects.

How can I tell if I'm at risk for depression?

Everyone is at risk for depression, just as you may be a possible target for almost any disease. But you're right if you think that some people are more at risk than others. It's not just because they have weaker personalities. The underlying culprits are a combination of genetic, chemical, and emotional risk factors:

- *Your DNA can put you at risk.* It is clear from a multitude of research that a tendency toward depression is inherited. Just as you are more likely to become prematurely bald if one or more members of your immediate ancestors lost their hair at an early age, you are more at risk for getting a mood disorder if someone in your family history has had it. The role of genetics becomes clear in studies on children adopted away from their natural parents who were known to have depression or manic depression. Enough of these children have shown increased vulnerability for depression (when compared to other children) in the adoptive home to suggest that the genes of their natural parents are more influential than environment. And, much research funded by the National Institute of Mental Health is now devoted to identifying genetic candidates that may fit the criteria as causal factors for depression and bipolar disorder.
- *A chemical impairment can put you at risk.* This could be some kind of inherited trait that affects the way your brain responds to emotional or physical stressors. Or, another type of chemical impairment can result from the effects of medication to treat high blood pressure or because of a thyroid problem. In fact, people with cancer, diabetes, stroke, or heart conditions have a noticeable risk of developing depression while their primary condition runs its course; up to 25 percent of people with those conditions will also subsequently develop depression. In some conditions, such as cancer of the pancreas or certain brain tumors, the risk of depression is even higher.
- *An emotional burden can put you at risk.* Even if someone

is not genetically inclined toward depression, the stresses involved in certain situations can still precipitate clinical depression. If some grief, loss, or humiliation is too heavy to bear, even healthy coping mechanisms can collapse. For example, you can see this in people who have a loved one who is suffering from a painful chronic disease or who were close to someone who committed suicide. In many cases, it is the combination of some stressor, a personal history of difficulties that have affected self-esteem or coping skills, and the lack of adequate support that trigger the onset of a depressive episode. Sometimes basic emotional makeup can contribute toward a depressive episode, too. For example, people who were shy as children appear to have a greater risk of subsequent depression. People with low self-esteem or a generally negative approach to situations are more likely to become overwhelmed by stress and develop clinical depression. In other cases, some severe early trauma, ongoing physical, sexual, or emotional abuse, or some other scarring event will alter our ability to tolerate stress permanently.

My sister doesn't suffer from depression but I do. How come, if there's a genetic connection?

On average, we share about 50 percent of the genes of each of our parents and each of our siblings. Why does one child inherit a grandmother's red hair while a sibling gets her coloring from a brown-haired father? Depression is another example of the genetic "draw." But depression is even more complicated than a random selection of genes. There are environmental and emotional factors at play, too. Look at it this way: There could be two people exposed to a cold virus— same virus, exposed the same way—but they may not both get colds. One person could be lucky enough to have naturally more antibodies to the virus. The other person may be tired and worn out from working for a demanding, unpleasant boss, and have less ability to fight off a virus at that moment in time. Or perhaps one, noting the exposure, took extra precautions, like dosing with zinc or, perhaps, vitamin C and getting plenty of rest that night. Luck's involved, too. The sneeze that sprays particles of the virus just doesn't happen to go up your nose or in your mouth, whereas it does to the other person. So developing a full-blown cold becomes a combination of individual vulnerability and coincidence.

I suffer from depression and so did my father. I'm worried about my sons. What early-warning signs should I be looking for?

A two-generation family history does suggest that your children have a higher risk, perhaps 2 or 3 times that of someone who has no ill relatives. But, even in the case of a single, powerful gene, each of your children would have no more than a 50 percent risk (if their other parent had no such risk). Whatever is happening in terms of such a gene, your children's developing sense of competence and self-esteem, exposure to environmental stressors, luck, and other factors (e.g., drug and alcohol abuse) are especially important. It is less common to see a child with onset of depression than an adult. If you think you see early warning signs (moodiness, social withdrawal, temper outbursts, crying spells, etc.) talk to your doctor or your child's pediatrician about your concerns.

If you fear a family gene, you can begin helping your child before depression shows up, by working with your toddler and growing child on developing good mechanisms for coping with problems. Many of these strategies can be incorporated into natural exchanges between parent and child, and some may even involve play. Some commonly noted:

- Encourage your child's sense of playfulness and fun
- Listen carefully to your child; you may miss depression's warning signs if you're not paying close attention
- Work on helping your child to relax; deep-breathing exercises are usually easy for children to master
- Reduce stresses in the home; protect your child from your own worries and problems

Learn "safe" ways for your child to express frustration, anger, and sadness—punching a pillow instead of a sibling, exorcising bad feelings through writing or physical activities, creating reward systems for good coping skills.

Creating an atmosphere of love, support and openness in your home will make it easier for a child to share fears and worries with you before they can mushroom into major problems. If there has been a history of frank, pressure-free discussion about depression in the household, appropriate to a child's age at any given time, it will make it easier for the adult that child will become to admit to the disorder if it ever develops and seek help.

There are other genetic factors involved, too. If a child has inherited or developed certain psychological traits, they may be at greater risk, simply because these characteristics make it harder to fend off depression's debilitating symptoms. So, yes, you should be more concerned if there's already a family gene and your child is persistently moody, reckless, shy, pessimistic, temperamental, fidgety, easily startled or frightened, impulsive, tempestuous, explosive, or has a tendency toward melancholy. Remember, though, that an occasional tantrum does not define a child as explosive, and a few weeks of low spirits after a pet dies is not necessarily melancholy.

If there is a genetic tendency toward depression, be alert for these signs, some of which mirror an adult's response to depression and others which are the slightly altered ways depression makes itself known in children:

- the school nurse reports frequent visits, and the child complains often of illnesses for which doctors can find no cause
- disturbances in sleep cycles
- a reluctance to talk that goes beyond shyness; the child appears sullen
- a generally tearful or worried demeanor
- persistent negative thoughts about himself, indicating low self-esteem
- weight loss or gain
- school attendance and grades drop
- runs away, or simply talks about it often

If these symptoms persist for more than two weeks, talk to your child's pediatrician and ask for a referral to a child psychologist. Always take suicidal statements seriously—children *can* kill themselves and teen suicide rates continue to increase.

There's no need for panic if depression is in your family history, though, just caution. Many people with a family history of the condition do not ever develop depression because they are able to establish healthy coping strategies to cover for possible genetic malfunctions. Likewise, people with no such history shouldn't think themselves immune to depression.

How can personality traits make you vulnerable if depression is a chemical imbalance, not a character flaw?

Again, the distinction between a chemical imbalance and a character flaw is a false one. For example, there is strong evidence of neurochemical alterations and hereditary factors in antisocial or sociopathic behavior and alcoholism. Why do two boys living in the same household go different routes when exposed to drugs—one becomes addicted, the other doesn't? How the drugs feel for one may be different from how they feel for the other, which is probably a biological reaction. But the perception of the pathway to success in life is also different and influences whether someone will succumb to the lure of the drug or seriously malfunction when depression strikes. Temperamental traits tell us things about our vulnerability in tandem with the neurochemical factors we do know about.

I don't have depression and, honestly, I can't even imagine what it's like. Is there any way you can make me understand what someone is feeling?

It's difficult to imagine this pain if you haven't experienced it. Still, I suppose the best and most basic way to describe depression is to say that it is all about struggle and not being able to have much control over things we take for granted (energy, sleep, appetite, sense of humor, etc). There are overwhelming self-doubts and a gnawing sense of pessimism and helplessness. When you are depressed, even the simplest decisions or activities can become an intense interior conflict; so painful and persistent a struggle that sometimes you can't muster the energy or the interest even to try. Think of it in these very simplistic terms:

As a healthy person, you might go to a movie feeling some sense of excited anticipation that the film would be a good one and that you would enjoy yourself. But let's say it turns out it was a real bomb, like *The Postman* or *Ishtar* and it was really very bad. If you're not depressed, your inclination is to blame the director or actors in a brief fit of pique. You might even ponder that you should have read a review or two before you saw the movie. But the meaning you would take away from all this would essentially be, "Well, I wasted eight bucks, but at least I get to trash the movie." You would come out of the experience with an explanation that didn't hurt you. And if you could share your disgust with a sympatico friend, all the better.

As a depressed person in the same situation, you would have expended greater exertion simply to get yourself to see the movie. First, you would have faced a more prolonged and distressing decision over whether it would be a waste of time. Then every minor inconvenience in getting there and finding a seat would have seemed to have justified your concern, and become almost insurmountable. And if the movie turned out to be a bomb, I'm pretty sure your interpretation of that bad movie would be something to the effect that, "This wasn't worth the effort. I knew it all along. I shouldn't have come here in the first place because nothing I do seems to make a difference." "I can't even pick out a good movie." The experience would become a painful focus on your own presumed failings and not those of the actors or film crew.

That's the kind of interior struggle a person in a major depressive episode faces down daily in all the small crises a normal day brings. From the most basic decisions like choosing between ice-cream brands and what to do when stuck in a traffic jam. Compounded by work conflicts, relationship questions, financial decisions, school pressures, the struggle becomes a war. Other sufferers use these words to describe it:

- "I feel like there's a wall between me and the rest of the world, and nothing positive can get past it."
- "It's like I'm reliving every bad experience of my life, every failure and rotten moment, over and over."
- "I can't seem to get my mind to shut off; everything that's making me worried or upset just keeps circling and circling around in my brain like some crazy rat running around on a wire wheel."
- "It's impossible to focus on anything; I try to concentrate but all these bad feelings rise up and get in the way."
- "There's this feeling of doom, like I know something

terrible is about to happen; nothing much ever does happen, but the feeling never ever goes away.''

Even though you can't conceive the pain, you can imagine the toll such constant struggle would take. Also, consider this toll, day in and day out, and the effect it would have on your morale. At some point, the future might seem so bleak that life doesn't seem worth living. This is when suicidal ideas begin to feel compelling. Continual emotional pain plus hopelessness is what drives self-destructive behavior.

Feeling the Effects of Depression

Let's say you can't comprehend the cost in pain—you can probably appreciate the damage in dollars. Here are some statistics that underscore the impact of depression:

Costs directly attributed to depression

Money spent on drugs and other pharmaceuticals	$1.2 billion
Outpatient or partial hospital care for treatment	$2.9 billion
Inpatient care for treatment	$8.3 billion
Money lost to decreased productivity of workers	$12.1 billion

(Disability from depression is more common than for any of the top 8 major diseases.)

Costs indirectly attributed to depression

Lost revenue caused by absenteeism	$11.7 billion

(This is in addition to decreased productivity—depression accounts for more employee sick days than hypertension, diabetes, or arthritis.)

continued

| Deaths, as a result of suicide | $7.5 billion |
| *Total estimated costs* | $43.7 billion |

*Based on estimates from a study by MIT and the Analysis Group.

Some organizations put the costs as even higher:

The National Institute of Mental Health (NIMH) credits mental disorders with a total cost of $150 billion each year for treatment, costs of social services, disability payments, lost productivity, and premature death, such as from suicides. The numbers are staggering.

When mental illness is treated, the results are equally impressive:

- $145 billion saved in the U.S. economy since 1970 from the treatment of manic-depressive disorder with lithium therapy
- $23,000 per patient per year saved on average by reducing hospital stays when schizophrenic patients use clozapine therapy
- $17,000 saved when people caring for family members who have Alzheimer's disease were placed in support programs; caretakers are typically hospitalized themselves with the stress responses of depression and fatigue
- 5 to 8 times the money spent on programs designed to diagnose and treat depression in elderly patients saved by these preventive measures, when hospital stays were cut by 2 days on average

I heard St. John's Wort works on depression that's "mild to moderate"? You mean you can rate depression?

An episode of depression can be rated for diagnostic purposes by the doctor/patient team, using a combination of recognized "scales." The patient describes his symptoms or is asked questions about them which help to assign a level of severity and track the frequency of episodes. This rating can influence the therapies chosen to fight the disorder, or just help to refine the diagnosis.

If, on the other hand, you wanted to compare the harshness of the various mood disturbances, you might rank them in an order like this, from bad to worse:

- a single episode of major depression
- recurrent major depression (repeated episodes)
- dysthymic disorder
- bipolar II (manic-depressive disorder with relatively brief highs)
- bipolar I (manic-depressive disorder with serious, out of control highs, associated with delusions, hallucinations, poor judgment)
- schizophrenia

Every year when winter rolls around, I get swamped by feelings of depression. What's happening?

It seems more and more people are becoming aware of this particular cycle of depressive illness—each year as winter arrives sufferers notice the recurring symptoms of fatigue, apathy, and a marked craving for foods high in carbohydrates. Weight gain, decreased sexual drive, extended sleep patterns, and a withdrawal from others are hallmarks of this seasonal cycle as well. If the episodes reach the severity of a full depressive syndrome, then the official diagnosis would be major depressive disorder, recurrent, seasonal pattern. More commonly, however, doctors and patients alike call this condition seasonal affective disorder, also known by its apt acronym, SAD. It is more often found in people who live in areas with four distinct seasons.

Of course, many people complain about simple, mild cases of "the winter blues"—it only enters the realm of mental illness when your response to the season is particularly marked and prolonged. In some people, the symptoms become debilitating. There is some thought that SAD may be tracked to depression's effects on the pineal gland, which regulates sleep cycles among its other hormone-related functions.

A physician can help determine whether your mood change is severe enough to be classified as seasonal affective disorder. Talk to your doctor about your condition to be sure it is not another form of depression, or based on some physical condition unrelated to depression. SAD often responds very well to a treatment that may seem incredibly natural: regular exposure to full-spectrum white light, a treatment called phototherapy. SAD may be, in fact, a malfunctioning physical response to fewer hours of sunlight. As with other forms of depression, your reaction to this stressor is not normal; it is excessive because your body's coping strategies are impaired in some way that is connected to light and sleep. Certainly, irregular melatonin and serotonin levels are probably implicated in SAD; the change in season appears to disrupt the essential cycles of our internal biological clock.

Ask for recommendations of treatments or products that can provide the light you need to beat SAD symptoms. Phototherapy sessions can be provided through your physician, but I have noticed a growing number of full-spectrum lamps cropping up in health-related consumer catalogs as well.

I hear people talk about being "bipolar." What is that?

You are probably more familiar with the term "manic-depressive," which is popularly used to describe this condition. It is a type of mood disorder which affects between 1 and 2% of the adult population. People who are bipolar can have wild mood swings, riding highs that can rival the height of Mount Everest and lows that resemble the depths of the Grand Canyon—the two "poles" on opposite ends of the emotional spectrum. The lows exhibit the classic symptoms of depression, and are labeled "depressive phase." Highs have the hallmarks of a state termed "mania" and are called "manic phase." Manic symptoms may include:

1. High energy levels with a feeling that there is less need for sleep (this feeling is false, of course, and the resultant insomnia can precipitate a fall from mania into depression)
2. Excitement, euphoria or anger which seems out of proportion to whatever stimulated it
3. Speech and actions that seem speeded-up
4. Overly quick decision-making, which leads to poor judgment (This can lead bipolar sufferers into financial difficulties and bad business decisions.)
5. More impulsive and potentially threatening sexual activity

6. Thoughts that race so fast it's difficult to articulate them; speech jumps from one subject to the next
7. Out-of-place or improper social behavior
8. An inflated sense of self-importance and feeling of power, resulting in grandiose ideas—when these ideas are consistently challenged by others paranoia may result, an extreme response to this perceived threat to the sufferer's false beliefs

In the movies, the flip-flop from one of these poles to the other is usually dramatically sudden. In reality, there are more often discrete, clear-cut episodes, with the period of mania lasting three months or even longer. There is often a period of normal mood and behavior ("euthymia" or the well-interval) between the poles and separating each cycle. But the pattern may repeat itself over and over until the bipolar sufferer gets help for the disorder. This type of depressive disorder is best treated with medication which helps stabilize the chemical shifts that drove the wild extremes.

Bipolar disorder typically has an earlier age of onset than unipolar, or recurrent major, depression. It is sometimes confused with schizophrenia, but is much more likely to be episodic as opposed to chronic, and doesn't usually involve the same deterioration of social behavior. Perhaps one-half of all bipolar sufferers could be considered "psychotic" in the sense that they are experiencing delusions or false beliefs about their wealth, power, talents, and attributes. Still, their actions are consistent with their delusions—if, say, a person believes that President Clinton has assigned them to some special post of honor, they would act in an appropriately excited and pleased way. This is distinct from schizophrenia, where a person may share a similar false belief but cannot react to even that with any kind of normal response. A person may sincerely believe President Clinton has named her Savior of the Human Race, but will tell you the news in a monotonous drone.

Sometimes the manic episode can persist until it literally exhausts the sufferer. Other times it can slide into a sustained state of psychosis. More often, though, the craziness of the manic phase feels exciting and euphoric as opposed to frightening. It's this infectious state of elation, creativity, and wild energy that has made the disorder oddly attractive to many people. The high number of writers, artists, entertainers, and sports figures that have openly acknowledged their disorder has also taken some of the sting from a diagnosis of this particular mental illness. The difficulty here is that while many sufferers want to keep the highs of their disorder, they uniformly wish to treat the lows—the depression which is bipolar's inevitable downside.

My sister has been diagnosed as schizophrenic. Her doctors used the term psychotic. All I can think about is all those old movies about nuts in insane asylums. How scared for her should I be?

You should be very concerned about your sister because schizophrenia is, sadly, the most chronic and disabling of all the mental disorders of young adult life. Anyone attempting to treat this disorder with an herbal remedy is wasting very precious time. Schizophrenia is not easily treated, and when someone with this illness recovers completely, there is good reason to question the diagnosis. There is a very high risk for suicide, so a quick and powerful response to the disorder is critical.

More than 2 million people in the U.S. may be diagnosed with schizophrenia in a given year; these sufferers are generally younger than those who experience mood disorders. Like bipolar disorder (also, at times, a "psychotic" illness), schizophrenia is marked by two kinds of warning signs, usually distinguished as "negative" and "positive" symptoms. Negative symptoms are more similar to major depression—a person withdraws from other people, can't communicate effectively, and experiences a dulling of all emotional responses. Positive symptoms, which do not justify their optimistic-sounding label, are the more obvious symptoms and those more popularly associated with the condition. These may include hallucinations (visions and voices) or delusions (believing in things that are patently untrue and not accepting evidence to the contrary). These may interact, so persons feel they are in communication with a higher, more powerful force which is influencing them and making them do things or feel a certain way. When these ideas are rebuffed the third or fourth time, delusions of persecution arise. Sometimes the hallucinations focus on the physical; persons may become convinced their stomach is infested with bugs.

Schizophrenia involves changes in the basic way one organizes thought. So, the schizophrenic not only experiences or believes things not in physical reality but the actual way she thinks and organizes thought is off-kilter. Usually what goes along with that over time is a gradual blunting or disinterest in the normal behaviors of a social animal. Attention to hygiene, dress, and other societal conventions declines rapidly. That's why so many people with schizophrenia are homeless or live in state hospitals or halfway houses. They just can't give a damn anymore about hygiene, schedules, etc.

As a family member of someone diagnosed with this severe and chronic disorder, the pressures may be intense enough to make you vulnerable to an episode of major depression yourself. Take care. Your sister's behavior is no doubt annoying and disruptive. You can only have the house set on fire so many times before, no matter how much you love her, she drives you to extreme responses yourself. That may seem a grotesque example, but bizarre and destructive behavior is not unusual in severe cases.

But there is hope. Researchers have made some amazing advances in the study of this disorder. They have used the newest brain-imaging techniques, such as MRIs and PET scans, to isolate what appears to be certain chemical abnormalities in the brain functions of people with schizophrenia. Some changes in biochemical responses have been observed that act as warning signs that the disorder may be present. This new information on the condition's causes will inevitably shed some light on its treatment. Your sister may find more options available to her soon.

In the meantime, you have taken the essential first step by seeking professional help and diagnosis. Now's the time to start asking questions. Share your concerns with your sister's physician. Her doctor should be aware of the toll this disorder takes on the whole family and should help guide you to support networks and programs that will strengthen your ability to cope with this thing. While St. John's Wort will not be able to help your sister, you certainly could discuss it with your doctor if you find yourself struggling with feelings of depression.

I keep getting these terrifying "fits"—my heart races, I sweat, start shaking, and feel like I'm going to have a heart attack. Am I crazy?

No, you are not crazy. You might be suffering from an actual cardiovascular condition, so I would be sure and see a physician to rule out common physical causes. But it is more likely that you've been experiencing panic attacks, one of several types of anxiety disorder.

Anxiety is the clinical companion of fear. Fear, in turn, is a necessary survival mechanism; healthy levels of this defense system has helped keep our species alive. Fear is a perfectly appropriate stress response to certain situations. It gets the body revved up to face some challenge or alerts you to possible danger. Everyone experiences anxiety at one point or another—the flip-flop in the stomach when a blind date rings the doorbell, the nervous tension and shakes if called on to give a speech, heart-pounding excitement before a race, even the adrenaline rush when sensing a threat. In appropriate doses, anxiety can help; it's a normal reaction. Anxiety *disorder*, however, is not normal. It is a crippling wave of nervous tension and distress which strikes at times when there is no apparent reason for anxiety. People with some form of the disorder may be aware, on a rational level, that there is nothing to provoke the response, but they will not be able to control their symptoms of worry or panic.

There are actually a number of subcategories of anxiety disorder recognized by the DSM-IV. While they all share the hallmark emotions of distress and dread, they seem to have chemical effects on different nerve centers, and thus have a variety of physical responses and are initiated by different psychological triggers:

Generalized Anxiety Disorder: chronic, excessive worry and tension that focus on anything (finances, work, relationships, health, school) or nothing (a general sense of impending disaster)

- GAD sufferers have problems slowing down their worrisome thoughts and relaxing or handling tension
- A host of physical symptoms may be present (tremors, twitching, sweating, headaches, muscle tension, shortness

of breath, dizziness, nausea, frequent urination, and insomnia)

Phobias: fear of very specific objects, situations and places; sufferers feel a total loss of control when confronted with the fear-object or a sense of being trapped

- The phobic response is more than extreme, it is completely irrational—often an individual knows this but is still unable to control the reaction

Panic Disorder: sudden, violent attacks of intense fear that strike without warning or apparent cause; the attack is generally accompanied by a sense of detachment from reality

- Attacks are marked by physical sensations of such intensity (dizziness, chills, numbness, sweating, the shakes, difficulty breathing, choking sensations, racing heart, and chest pain), a person feels as if she is about to die or is losing his mind
- Panic attacks can wake a person from a sound sleep
- Episodes are usually of short duration, 1 to 10 minutes, but in rare instances may last up to an hour
- Agoraphobia is a frequent companion of panic disorder; it is a fear of being somewhere you cannot escape from or hide when a panic attack strikes. The name comes from Greek (fear of the market place) and basically describes a person who has become ''housebound'' because of his or her fears

Post-Traumatic Stress Disorder (PTSD): a condition which follows exposure to a severe trauma—a psychologically terrifying, physically stressful, or otherwise disturbing event (military actions, disasters, plagues, physical attacks, accidents, witnessing a violent act)

- PTSD is noticeably worse when related to an event initiated by a person (such as a terrorist attack, rape, or kidnapping), rather than a natural disaster
- Symptoms include flashbacks that relive the trauma; a numbness or intellectual distancing from both the original event and people close to you; sleep disturbances; loss of

appetite; disinterest in sex; trouble expressing affection; increased tendency toward rage or violence; the capacity to be easily startled or frightened
- PTSD used to be called shell shock or battle fatigue when observed in war veterans
- Symptoms are considered "normal" stress responses for up to a month after the initiating event, recognized as a mental disorder when symptoms persist in intensity beyond that period
- Psychotherapy and/or medication is necessary to help address this persistent and disabling disorder; a strong support network can make recovery much faster

Obsessive-Compulsive Disorder (OCD): a focus on some insignificant or imagined detail to an extent so habitual and unwavering it is no longer rational

- The fixed thoughts are "obsessions," the ritualistic actions associated with them are "compulsions"
- Obsessions may be disturbing thoughts and images which appear and reappear endlessly, i.e. a sufferer may suddenly recall that she was born on a Tuesday and become convinced that she will therefore die on a Tuesday, fearing each week's approach of that day with a manic terror
- Compulsions often present as bizarre, time-consuming routines such as a need to touch or count things, i.e., numbering every square of the sidewalk each time you walk the street or consistently performing every menial action in sets of 3 because that's arbitrarily chosen as a lucky number
- Obsessions and compulsions become so important nothing else seems to matter

Again, repetition, unprovoked, persistent is the key to the diagnosis of these anxiety disorders, since many people will experience some kind of extreme anxiety response at least once in their lifetimes, the result of a temporary overburdening of normally healthy coping mechanisms.

Antidepressant medications are sometimes effective in alleviating some of the symptoms of anxiety disorder, but treatment more often involves a combination of drugs and behavioral therapies (more on these in the following chapter). While St. John's Wort may have an effect on milder cases of anxiety, it's thought to have little influence on full-fledged OCD, agoraphobia, or PTSD, and would be of little use in the midst of a panic attack.

Is there a connection between anxiety and depression?

Anxiety disorders seem to have some link to depression, if only because people with anxiety disorders often develop major depression if their initial condition is left untreated. The connection may be as simple as cause and effect, or impaired responses to different aspects of the same stressor. I think of this connection as that of threat and loss, for instance: the threat of a parent's dying, as a result of a mother's diagnosis with cancer, might produce classic GAD symptoms. If that parent were to die, then the threat has materialized into a genuine loss, and a vulnerability to depression is created.

How does a doctor figure out which kind of problem I have?

Doctors use a set of criteria developed by the American Psychiatric Association to identify and classify your illness: *The Diagnostic and Statistical Manual of Mental Disorders*, more fondly referred to as the DSM. Regularly updated to reflect the latest psychiatric findings, it lists 25 different broad categories and over 100 subcategories of mental illness, then identifies the recognized symptoms for each. Some of the categories that would be more familiar to you are listed in the chart on page 68.

Armed with this reference, a doctor might also use a variety of tests, including blood workups and brain scans to pinpoint any potential physical causes for your symptoms, and ask you questions designed to develop a full health and family history. You'll be asked about current and past symptoms, will discuss their severity, and look at how they were treated. Any problems with substance abuse must be shared in order to target your treatment most effectively. Careful probing will help reveal if other members of the family have displayed similar symptoms, to discover whether a clear genetic tendency may exist. Your doctor will ask if you have ever considered suicide. This body of information will combine to point to a diagnosis.

Recent research into biochemical changes recorded in people suffering from a variety of mental illnesses suggests that we also may be able to use sophisticated neuroimaging techniques, like PET scans (positron emission topography) and MRI (magnetic resonance imaging) measuring brain activity, to distinguish between the different disorders.

Since the adoption of the uniform criteria listed in the DSM, diagnosis has become far more reliable and consistent; for example, the diagnoses of major depressive disorder and bipolar disorder are made with the accuracy levels at or above other areas of medicine.

Selected Categories from *The Diagnostic and Statistical Manual of Mental Disorders*

Anxiety Disorders
    phobias
    panic disorder
    post-traumatic stress disorder (PTSD)
    obsessive-compulsive disorder (OCD)
Mood Disorders
    major depression
    manic-depressive disorder
Schizophrenia
Disruptive Behavior Disorder
    attention deficit hyperactivity disorder (ADHD)
    conduct disorder
Substance Abuse Disorders
    alcoholism
    drug dependence
Delusional Disorders
    delusional paranoia
Sexual Disorders
Sleep Disorders
Dissociative Disorders
    multiple-personality disorders
Eating Disorders
    anorexia
    bulimia

I talk about feeling stressed all the time. But what does that word really mean? Is it the same thing as depression?

In the psychiatric world, "stress" is a term describing any type of physical or mental strain that, in excess, can result in measurable pathological results. That simply means that any factor in your physical or social environment and mental or emotional makeup that provokes a response is called a stressor. And the responses you have to these factors—feelings of tension, worry, and fear—are labeled stress. In the nonmedical world, people commonly use the single word "stress" to mean both these things.

The more extreme the stress, then, the more extreme a response: a terrible wound (stressor) might permit a dangerous infection (stress) if the body's functions fail to cope with the harmful bacteria, a job loss (stressor) which leads to financial difficulties (stressor) might provoke feelings of deep anxiety and confusion (stress) if your coping mechanisms aren't able to function effectively with that situation. In a chain reaction, the stress then helps sets the stage for depression.

So, how much stress is *too* much? It depends on the unique personality and mental health of the individual. Healthy people are equipped with mechanisms for handling a great deal of stress, at least for temporary periods. But people who have depression disorder have coping mechanisms that don't function as well as a healthy person's might, so the stress response is far more profound. And because stress has both physical and mental impacts, if it is sustained, the depressed person's entire system is affected. Regular sleep cycles are one of the first to go.

Some studies indicate that stresses play a particularly significant role in precipitating the first episode of major depression. But a third or fourth episode and those that follow are much less likely to be related to any discernible stressor. It seems that once stress has pried open the door—once a pattern has been established—nothing more is really needed to invite depression in.

Why is this happening now?

Sometimes a person with a tendency toward depression is launched into a full-scale depressive episode as a result of a single event—a death in the family, a job loss, school pres-

sures, a love affair gone sour. That event, while not the root
cause of the depression, acts like the straw that broke the
camel's back. Piled on top of already low feelings, a genetic
tendency toward the condition, and a coping mechanism that
isn't functioning, the event is simply too much to handle. This
is especially true of situations and conditions which alter sleep
patterns and other regular body rhythms such as eating patterns
or menstrual cycles.

Still, for many people with a mood disorder there is no
specific event that would seem to spur the depression. This
type of depression is sometimes known as endogenous depression, meaning its onset originates from something happening within the patient not in response to some outside stimulus.
Of course, there may be a physical "event" at play that you
are not consciously aware of; some of these associated with
depression involve a shift in hormone levels, like puberty or
menopause.

**I just surfaced from an episode of major depression. It was
pretty bad, but I made it through without help. Tell me
this will never happen again.**

I can't tell you that. The sad fact is that just the opposite is
true. People who have had one major depressive episode in
their lifetime have at least a 50 percent chance and perhaps a
70 percent lifetime chance of a subsequent depression, without
some type of continuing treatment. Moreover, during the first
few months of feeling better people are at a high risk to relapse
without ongoing treatment. If repeated new episodes are diagnosed, the disorder is further defined as recurrent major depressive disorder.

And now for some more bad news . . . What may not occur
again is the ability to "get through" the next episode without
help. The people who have the best chance of getting better
without any treatment or with relatively weaker therapies, like
St. John's Wort, are people in milder episodes, perhaps most
especially during the first episode of depression—partly because people in their first episode have the best chance of
getting better, period. As the number of lifetime episodes begins to add up, though, the signs and symptoms of the depression begin to change. With successive episodes the
disorder can become more and more severe. It can develop

into chronic depression in about one in four cases if left untreated. There is often less confusion about diagnosis for these later episodes, as the depression generally becomes less understandable from the grief or stress model. After a few episodes no event may be needed to trigger an attack. If you struggled with your first episode, I would strongly suggest confirming a diagnosis with a doctor, discussing any appropriate preventive measures, and working on developing even more efficient coping mechanisms.

Of course, that "50–70 percent relapse" figure means there is a subset of people who become significantly depressed once in their lifetimes, get better, and are never hit with it again. I hope you are one of them.

Lately, I've been feeling intense rage at everyone and everything. People tell me I'm reacting way out of proportion. Could it be depression?

A change in behavior can be linked to physical diseases and other conditions besides depression, so see a doctor to get an accurate diagnosis. Your sudden shift in mood may be linked to a mental disorder, other than depression; yet another reason to get your diagnosis clarified by a professional. Depressed and anxious men are more likely to express their symptoms through affects of anger and present them through physical violence than women, perhaps a result of cultural imperatives. Or the link between rage and depression may have something to do with levels of serotonin. The neurotransmitter may help control behaviors clinically labeled as "impulsive"—fury, injury to self and others. In studies, people with lower-than-normal levels of serotonin were observed to be more likely to express depression impulsively.

My doctor tells me I'm suffering from depression. But I don't feel sad, just kind of detached and disinterested in things.

Ironically, the feeling of depression or sadness is not always the most marked emotion of someone suffering from depression disorder. A lack of interest in activities that were once pleasurable or meaningful is a common hallmark of the disorder. Some people simply feel numb, with little or no emotional reaction whatsoever. These responses might be accompanied by sadness, but often they overwhelm even that emotion. In terms of its effects, apathy can be just as disabling a response as despair. Still, if you feel doubtful about a diagnosis, talk to your doctor about how and why it was made. If you can't get a satisfactory answer, see another physician for a second opinion.

I've been diagnosed with depression disorder. But I don't have the symptoms I hear about—in fact the opposite. What's up?

You may have a type of depression that is sometimes called "atypical depression," despite the fact that it is actually quite common. This classification is recognized as a subform of major depression and dysthymia. I assume that you're talking about symptoms that don't seem to fit into the classic list: Instead of loss of appetite, consumption of food is increased; rather than insomnia, a person experiences prolonged episodes of sleep. A person with atypical depression can still find pleasure in certain activities. Atypical depression is most common among younger patients, especially young women diagnosed with depression. Of course, there is also the possibility that your doctor is not correct, so ask why the diagnosis of depression was made.

What other disease or disorder has symptoms that can be confused with those of depression?

A number of diseases and disorders share symptoms commonly associated with depression. Diabetes, thyroid disorders, or chronic high blood pressure are those most commonly cited. But there are many others, among them: chronic upset stomach and other digestive disorders, migraine, nutritional deficiencies or a poor diet, mononucleosis, hypoglycemia, endometriosis, lead poisoning and toxic reactions to other heavy metals, or allergies. Some of the conditions that mimic depression can be quite serious, while others are easily treated once they have been identified—two very good reasons to share your symptoms and concerns with a physician instead of trying to self-diagnose your condition.

Are there health problems that contribute to depression or put you more at risk?

Absolutely. Any kind of disease or disability makes you more vulnerable to depression. Technically, any condition that affects quality of life doubles your lifetime's chance for depression—arthritis or diabetes or a learning disability—anything which adds difficulty to your life and greater risk for adversity, loss, and setbacks could increase your chances for depression, even if there is no family tendency toward the disorder.

In addition to conditions such as AIDS that precipitate depression because of the physical and mental stresses involved, there are diseases that put you at risk because they target specific areas of the brain or hormones. Infections like influenza, viral hepatitis, mononucleosis, and tuberculosis can also provoke a depressive response. Brain tumors and other neurological diseases, certain thyroid disorders, and hormonal conditions like Cushing's disease, can all take you over and above the liability model, too. In other words, these conditions first have something in their chemistry which alters the brain's function and makes you more likely to get depression, and then their disabling physical effects make you increasingly vulnerable to the disorder. The risk for depression instead of being doubled becomes quadrupled in those cases. Parkinson's disease and some cardiovascular conditions have a greater chance of provoking depression than other illnesses similar in severity and physical impact. Some sort of chemical connection seems indicated, but we're not sure exactly what it is.

Cancer patients are very vulnerable to depression. Cancer cells are cells out of control, and they can produce chemical substances humans don't ordinarily make. One particular cancer, located at the head of the pancreas, makes it sufferers twice as likely to develop depression than do other cancers of the abdomen. In fact, depression can present before other symptoms with that condition. That particular cancer is producing something that fosters the disease; it is what we call a depressogenic agent.

Not surprisingly, it works the other way, as well. Studies suggest that patients suffering a life-threatening illness who then develop depression are 5 times more likely to experience complications or die from their disease. This number can be significantly affected if the depression is successfully treated.

Everyone I know who's been diagnosed with depression is a woman. Is this a "woman's disease"?

The statistics, if taken out of context, look like this: lifetime prevalence for all depressive disorders is as high as 10 to 16 percent for women, while only 5 to 8 percent for men. Some argue that these numbers don't reflect the true picture, that men are less apt to seek treatment for their condition and so are not fully represented in the roll or that their symptoms are more likely to be misdiagnosed as some more socially "legitimized" disease. Still, it seems clear there is some sort of connection. What is the connection? Now that is an interesting question and one hotly debated issue. Here are the two basic camps:

It's about hormones: If hormones are the one of the biggest chemical culprits behind depression, then you can see why there is such a strong connection between women and depression. A woman's hormonal cycles experience more dramatic and distinct shifts throughout her life, although hormonal shifts in men, while less visible, also occur. The increased risks for depression associated with the use of oral contraceptives (the Pill), pregnancy, childbirth, premenstrual syndrome and menopause are well documented. In addition, women are more likely to develop some thyroid conditions known to precipitate depression. Estrogen and progesterone have been linked to the functions of the hypothalamus, the control center for body functions that follow regular patterns, like sleep and menstrual cycles. Higher levels or abrupt shifts in the amounts of the two hormones may disturb the hypothalamus's delicate balance and increase vulnerability to mental disorders which seem so closely tied to such circadian rhythms.

It's about social roles and pressures: Other researchers believe hormones are only a small part of the picture, that social factors are the major factors behind the significant gender differences for depression and anxiety disorders. They cite women's greater exposure to certain stressors—noting they are more likely to be the victims of physical violence or infidelity; to experience job loss or be overlooked for promotion and power; and act as the caregiver to chronically ill family members—all well-known depression stressors. And, just when scientists are about to make sweeping statements about the correlation between hormones and mental illness, they are brought up short by the anomalies: for instance, the statistics for bipolar disorder are much closer to a 50–50 split. And some studies of depression conducted in Amish communities, where social influences like spousal abuse, infidelity, and divorce are almost nonexistent, demonstrate depression numbers with a much slimmer gender gap. So cultural stressors and strong support networks may play as much of a role as hormones or counteract their damaging effects.

One factor that bridges these camps is the difference in how men and women characteristically cope with strong emotions. Whereas men are more likely to use distraction and active, action-oriented coping strategies, women are better at emotion-focused coping methods. These stereotypes, which of course don't characterize all men and women, may actually correspond to sex differences in how the brain hemispheres process different emotions. Such differences may help to reinforce traditional roles (hunter-gatherer versus caregiver) that aren't as relevant in modern, western life. Thus, we live in a world far different that the one our brain is adapted to and the brunt of these differences falls disproportionately on women.

Until we know more, however, it hurts everyone to label any form of mental illness a "woman's" or "man's" disease. Doing so will hamper some people from ever seeking help for their conditions, because they fear societal scorn or rejection. It can also blind some doctors to diagnosis, those who continue to look for other causes for symptoms when a history makes it clear where the true cause lies.

I feel like crying all the time, and when I'm alone I just fall apart. Could this be related to my recent pregnancy?

A high number of pregnant women and recent mothers experience some feelings of depression immediately after having their babies. They present the common symptoms of mild depression: persistently low mood, loss of self-esteem, irritability, and anxiety. Crying jags are a natural release of these bad feelings. A temporary depression at this time is perfectly normal and typically not reason for concern. After all, a woman's body has just gone through tremendous physical stress, and the responsibilities of new parenthood can be enough to provoke temporary feelings of depression in anyone. In addition, a new mother's body is coping with a radical shift in the levels of hormones it has been producing for months; this sudden decrease in estrogen and progesterone can precipitate mood swings, hair loss, breakouts of acne, and more severe bouts of PMS. If that isn't enough to depress someone getting up every four hours through the night, I'm not sure what is.

Normally, however, the body adjusts to the physical changes and new demands, a mother bonds with her child so that the rewards of parenthood begin to outweigh its stresses. The temporary letdown and anxiety pass. For those few weeks of low moods, though, St. John's Wort might be an option—providing your physician approves its use if you are breast-feeding (no studies have been done of the herb's effects on nursing infants).

The key word for a normal reaction, however, is "temporary," just as it is in other types of depression. While a period of moodiness following delivery is often casually referred to as postpartum depression, it only really deserves that name when it becomes a true disorder—when the changes in mood continue for more than a few weeks or become disabling. The new mother is overwhelmed by her feelings of depression and has trouble getting through a wide range of daily activities, including care of the infant. Sometimes depressed mothers struggle with overpowering feelings of anger toward the baby, and these can put the child at risk. Needless to say, it is imperative to get help in treating your depression if you begin to experience intense fury and frustration, to protect both your child and yourself.

Do not resign yourself to holding it all in until you are alone. Your condition will only get worse when you isolate yourself and don't get the help you need to get better. Share your worries and feelings with your family. They are probably more aware of your struggle than you know. Discussing your depression could be a relief for everyone. And talk to your doctors about your feelings, right away. If it isn't a true episode of postpartum depression, your doctor may have suggestions for speeding the normal recovery process. If it is a case of clinical postpartum depression, the disorder typically responds well to treatment, although options besides drug therapy have to be considered if the new mother is nursing. If your primary-care physician is dismissive of your symptoms, even after a number of weeks have passed, talk to your gynecologist, who will be more familiar with the disorder. If that doctor is unresponsive as well, insist on being referred to a psychiatrist or psychologist, or consider switching to a new physician who will take you seriously. It's a sad fact that postpartum depression is often shrugged off by doctors as simply a phase. But no phase should last very long or be disabling. This condition is a recognized psychiatric disorder and should be treated that way.

My doctor calls my insomnia a "hallmark" of depression. What's that mean?

Your doctor is referring to the fact that persistent insomnia is a classic symptom of depression, and in your case might be one of the more distinct or problematic of those symptoms. Most people occasionally have a night or two of sleeplessness, times when they can't shut their minds down. The seriously depressed person can't *ever* shut down his or her mind. You can imagine the toll this must take on sleep patterns.

Healthy people have the capacity to lose part of a night's sleep, even several nights', without too much cost to overall well-being. This temporary sleeplessness may be the result of worry or excitement. But too much lost sleep and even a healthy person pays the price: Attention and concentration diminish, motor functions falter, and your immune system becomes weakened. A depressed person loses sleep to insomnia night after night after night. Soon, in addition to other symptoms of depression, an individual must cope with the additional burden of the results of this sleeplessness. It can become too much to bear without help.

Sleep disturbances in depressed patients can present themselves in a variety of ways besides what's commonly thought of as insomnia: problems falling asleep, frequent awakenings throughout the night, waking excessively early, sleeping very late, drowsiness during the day. In sleep studies of depressed patients, a quicker slide into the REM (rapid eye movement) stage of sleep and odd patterns in that normally regularly cycled phase were noted. REM is the period in which a person dreams, and during which certain motor functions are inhibited. Melatonin and serotonin levels are affected during various sleep stages (you'll find more on these chemicals elsewhere in the chapter).

Why do depressed people have so much trouble with sleep cycles? We know depression strikes at glands which regulate an array of body rhythms including sleep. There may be some alteration in the signals controlling sleep patterns, perhaps messages become less intense. Or maybe there's a defective way of dampening or softening the signals, so they are always the same strength. Thoughts are then never slowed down enough to allow sleep. Perhaps something is blocking the pathways that translate environmental information to the brain, messages like "it's dark" and "it's light," which can interfere with sleep. We don't know for sure what the exact culprit may be.

Is chronic fatigue syndrome a form of depression?

Chronic fatigue syndrome, or CFS, is not a psychiatric illness. Instead, CFS is believed to be the result of an altered immune response to viral infection. Until recently Epstein-Barr was thought to be the likely viral source but now it's believed EBV may *result* from CFS, not the other way around. There is sometimes confusion about CFS and its relationship to depression, because the disease shares some of the same symptoms classically associated with psychiatric illness, such as very low energy levels and fatigue so persistent and debilitating it inspired the syndrome's name. Feelings of depression might be one of the syndrome's symptoms, but depression is not the root cause of the condition. CFS is distinguished from depression by various flulike and neurological symptoms such as sore throat, digestive troubles, and swollen lymph nodes. Some bodies react to the disease by going into immune overdrive, producing excessive immune responses that lead to joint and muscle pain, as well as headaches. Other bodies respond the opposite way, by suppressing the immune response. Because the symptoms vary, and many are similar to those of a number of other diseases, CFS is often difficult to identify, and misdiagnoses, including depression, are still common. There is not yet any test for the disease, so other potential sources of the symptoms must be eliminated, leaving CFS as the only option. There is no known cure for the condition, so its symptoms are addressed instead, with painkillers and antidepressants, which simply adds to the confusion surrounding the disease's relationship to depression.

How are some digestive upsets related to depression?

Currently, there is investigation into the causes and precise symptoms of a condition now known as functional bowel disorder. This term is being applied to a collection of common, chronic, and occasionally disabling gastrointestinal disorders. This collection of disorders, which includes irritable bowel syndrome, may affect up to 18 percent of the population and particularly targets women, who make up between 70 and 90 percent of those presenting with its array of symptoms. These may encompass anything from simple bloating to difficult or irregular bowel movements, painful constipation, or abdominal pain.

Whether this condition's symptoms are linked to depression is still not known, but it is sometimes mentioned in relation to mood disturbance. Perhaps it is a particular kind of physical response to depression or a disorder experienced congruent with depression, one that is vulnerable to the same stressors as the mood disorder.

What is the relationship between depression and alcoholism?

They are obviously related in the basic sense that both are mental disorders—depression is a mood disorder and alcoholism a substance abuse disorder. But these conditions share more than just neighboring spots on some diagnostic chart. The risk that a chemically dependent person will develop depression in his lifetime may be higher than 50 percent. The converse is also true—it has been noted that people with major depression run about twice the risk for alcoholism and other substance abuse than nondepressed people. They typically choose chemicals that seem temporarily to quiet or dampen depression's pain, such as alcohol, sedatives, nicotine, or marijuana. What's more, the families of clinically depressed people also run a higher risk for substance abuse.

When depression and addiction share the stage, the resultant tangle is called "dual disorder." By the time most people who suffer from this dual disorder seek treatment, the primary problem is the addiction. It takes on a life of its own. Taking care of that is the highest priority. Everything else is blocked by the addiction and can't be addressed until that blocking force has been eliminated.

Even if you do not abuse them, some drug therapies can increase your risk for depression, too, especially if a person has a family history of mental illness. This may be caused by the drug's actions on enzymes, hormones, or neurotransmitters (more about these chemicals follows), or because of some less-definable chemical link to depression. See the list below for some of the culprits.

If You Are Genetically Vulnerable to Depression, Ask Your Doctor About the Risks in Taking . . .

amantadine
amphetamines
antineoplastic (cancer-fighting) drugs
benzodiazepines (when abused)
beta-blocking drugs (not all are linked to depression)
birth-control pills
carbazepine
chloral hydrate
clonidine
cocaine
cycloserine
digitalis
disulfiram
estrogen and progesterone (any ERT therapies)

haloperidol
hydralazine
indapamide
indomethacin
levodopa
methyldopa
opiates
pentazocine
phenthiazines (not all are linked to depression)
physostigmine
prazosin
quanethidine
reserpine
steroids (those chemically similar to cortisone)
succinimide derivatives
sulfonamides

So now I know about depression. But what I really want to know is why is it happening to *me*?

Genetics. Job loss. Financial troubles. Chronic physical pain. Malfunctioning neurotransmitters. A bad breakup. Overactive enzymes. A death in the family. A poor family relationship. Daily trips on the freeway. Any, all, or none of these might be a reason it is happening to you. That isn't intended to be flip. The truth is we're simply not sure exactly why depression or other mental illnesses are happening at all, just that all of these things may play roles, along with many other chemical, emotional, and environmental factors. But we can say that mental illness is not the result of something bad you have done or some kind of character flaw. If the flaw exists, it is in your basic chemical makeup, not in your character. And in scientific or medical terms that can only be credited to a random mix of DNA.

Why should I care about depression?

In 1996, suicide was listed as one of the top ten leading causes of death, right up there beside cancer, heart disease, and accidents. But suicide is no accident, and depression is the most common factor in all suicides—*all* of them across the board in all age groups. More than half of depressed people will attempt suicide if their disorder is left untreated. A distressing 17 percent of them will succeed in taking their lives. The emotional toll and financial costs not just to the sufferers but to the whole society are tremendous. And don't forget the depressives who turn their pain and anger outward, toward others, rather than against themselves. Even if you had no more personal connection to depression, you could become a victim of that aspect of the disorder. Everyone should care about this condition, and about the new therapies, like St. John's Wort, that might be used successfully to treat it. The condition is saddening, but the apathy and ignorance expressed toward it, and the numbers of victims left untreated, are simply maddening.

I have been diagnosed as clinically depressed. And yet I still don't know what to say when people tell me it's not normal to react this way to stress.

Next time, respond by telling them they're right. Depression is an *abnormal* reaction, not a normal one, which is precisely why it is an illness. Diabetes is not a normal reaction to blood sugar. A heart attack is not a normal reaction to blood pressure. But they are inevitable responses for a body that does not have the ability to cope with blood sugar or blood pressure because of some biological malfunction.

As someone with clinical depression, you have a biological dysfunction that provokes an emotional response similar to the physical responses created by those other conditions—some kind of biochemical breakdown that does not allow parts of your brain to react to stress in a way that is considered normal. Just because no one knows yet exactly why this happens or what specific biochemical is to blame does not make it any less a legitimate disorder. No one knows precisely what causes cancer, yet people do not question that illness's legitimacy, or wonder why people don't just "cope" with it. Cancer is not a normal physical reaction; treatment is required to stop it from physically destroying its host. Depression is not a normal reaction; treatment is needed to stop it from mentally destroying *its* host.

Only through education will depression lose its stigma as a character flaw and be recognized as the illness it truly is. Luckily, more and more is becoming known about mental illness, and, gradually, this information is working its way through the clouds of confusion. Cultural icons are admitting to the disorder; admittedly, this is occasionally a ploy for attention in a crowded media, but it still focuses a spotlight on mental illness and sheds a little light on the subject. As a result, there is no question that fewer negative associations are attached to both depression and its therapy than was the case a generation ago.

Still, uninformed comments remain common. Don't wait for the next media breakthrough to educate your friends and family. Share what you know about depression and other forms of mental illness. If you don't know the basics yourself, read this chapter to find out more. If you have trouble explaining the condition, use the literature. Get more information from the organizations listed in the resource chapter. You'll be able to respond more effectively to remarks like those from people ignorant of the facts.

My wife's been told she's clinically depressed. She was never a weak person before—why can't she handle things anymore?

First of all, you should know that words like "strong" or "weak" are very judgmental terms that can have a tremendous negative impact on someone suffering with depression. The disorder predisposes people to think in discrete black and white categories. So, if someone they care about picks pejorative terms to describe them, like weak, worthless, or helpless, they'll accept that picture of themselves. Try to be careful about the language you use in discussions about this disorder, because self-esteem is one of the first victims of depression. You could be taking a whack at someone who's already down.

Next, ask yourself: Was Winston Churchill a weak person? Was Abe Lincoln? Martin Luther? Oliver Cromwell? Theodore Roosevelt? There is good documentation to support the claim that these men all suffered from depression disorder. Others have achieved amazing accomplishments in spite of their condition, including influential political figures like Queen Elizabeth, Boris Yeltsin, and Barbara Bush; creative adepts such as Kurt Vonnegut, Leonard Cohen, Ernest Hemingway, Sandra Cisneros, Lou Reed, and James Taylor; and sports or entertainment icons like Francis Ford Coppola, Dwight Gooden, Monica Seles, Greg Louganis, Dolly Parton, Mike Wallace, and Rod Steiger. These people all had a vulnerability, but no one's calling them weak personalities. Yet they all are or were depressed.

Depression is not a question of moral strength, but of chemistry and a breakdown of coping mechanisms. In fact, if you take away anything from this chapter, it should be perhaps not so much what depression is as what it is *not*:

- Depression is *not* just the result of a personality flaw or a weakness of character. It is *not* about a lack of willpower or gumption.
- Mental illness is *not* something that will go away on its own—this episode may end, but another is almost certain to follow if left untreated.

- Depression is *not* a strictly emotional state; it's got a bio-chemical factor that can't be willed away no matter how strong a person may be.
- A depressed person is *not* nuts or inherently unstable; with treatment, a depressed person can be made well enough to handle all of life's daily struggles and crises.
- Mental illness is *not* something you can cause by some kind of bad behavior or emotional trait. Depression affects behavior or takes advantage of traits but is not caused by these factors.
- Depression is *never* "your fault." Its cause is beyond your control. But its treatment isn't. You can always do something to help yourself.

THREE

❦

Conventional Treatment of Depression

This book is about St. John's Wort. However, it is also about depression. And any discussion of the two really must also address the conventional treatment options available for mood disorder, to give you a complete picture of how the herbal remedy might fit into the bigger picture of depression treatment. This chapter will provide answers to the most common questions about those other options, including antidepressant medications and psychotherapies. With the facts in hand, you'll be better armed to weigh their known pros and cons against those of St. John's Wort.

At this still-uncertain stage in St. John's Wort's use as a depression therapy in the U.S., my recommendation is to consider this herb an experimental treatment. Perhaps a word or two about this notion will make my position clearer. I do not, for example, mean that no one should take St. John's Wort unless they are in a formal scientific study. I do think that there are several facts that should be considered before rushing out to the health food store. First, depression can be a serious illness and even its milder forms can have negative effects on one's work and family life. Second, there are many types of antidepressant medications and several forms of psychotherapy that have been shown to be effective in well-controlled studies. Third, although the European studies are promising, St. John's Wort has not been studied with the same rigor as these alternate treatments. And fourth, St. John's Wort is not manufactured with the same quality control and standardization as the

FDA-approved antidepressants. "Natural" is not necessarily better (e.g., arsenic and cobra venom are natural, too!).

It *is* clear that St. John's Wort has generally mild side effects and that the major danger of self-prescription is delay of obtaining an accurate diagnosis and standard treatment. It therefore *should not* be chosen if you are suicidal, incapacitated, or under marked pressure to get better quickly. By the way, these suggested restrictions are similar to the ones we use to decide who is eligible to participate in placebo-controlled studies of new antidepressants. Of course, the herb is primarily being eyed by those sufferers who aren't so impaired and who haven't ever considered using the more widely accepted therapies for depression—millions who have yet to receive *any* kind of treatment for this disorder at all. So, for this group, I believe that St. John's Wort is a viable option as long as the costs and potential benefits are understood, response is monitored carefully, and alternate treatments are again considered if the herb is not helpful within four to six weeks.

Why don't more people get treatment? It's due to a combination of factors involving both patients and their doctors. In the case of the depression sufferers themselves, it may be attributed to the simple fact that many don't even recognize that their symptoms constitute a recognized disorder. They may not ever visit a physician for their symptoms (i.e., fatigue or insomnia), and so never learn these symptoms can be treated. A few people may not have access to treatment facilities because of location or lack of transportation. More commonly, treatment is available but perceived to be too difficult—too many roadblocks. Even if people are aware of treatment options, they may know only their side effects or harbor false beliefs about their dangers, as news media seize on negative stories as a way to grip interest and place an exaggerated focus on the downside of some treatments. Fear of society's reaction and stigma is another reason behind undertreatment of depression. People are afraid to admit to the misunderstood disorder or talk about its symptoms. Again, there is the old bias that depression is a sign of weakness and treatment is a "cop-out."

Sometimes, doctors are at fault. Some primary-care providers have too little education about depression; even a specialist in internal medicine may have had poor training or not kept up-to-date. Some doctors frequently misdiagnose or fail to recognize depression's symptoms, especially those of chronic depression. Some doctors are unable to communicate effectively with patients about the condition in a way that encourages treatment. And now in the era of managed care, many physicians can't spend enough time with a patient to note symptoms or fully explain them. A seven- to ten-minute office visit doesn't permit much time for exploration! Doctors who don't know their patients well may suggest treatments their patients wouldn't consider, without exploring options or taking the time to demystify misunderstood therapies.

As a result of all these complications, far too many cases go untreated, by conventional therapies as well as alternative. More than half of the people suffering from depression disorder will obtain no treatment that focuses on their disorder; nearly 40% of those who suffer from bipolar disorder will go similarly untreated.

Complicating matters is the regrettable fact that some health-care practitioners have relatively fixed treatment philosophies which they can defend with great prejudice against all comers, friend or foe. All the various disciplines are guilty of this—biologically-oriented psychiatrists, psychoanalysts, "growth"-oriented counselors, addiction specialists, behavioral psychologists, even naturopaths, homeopaths, and herbalists. That's a shame, because research has shown that if one form of therapy for depression doesn't work well within two to three months, it doesn't help matters to continue it longer. If a therapy isn't generating a response after 8–12 weeks, it is time to investigate options or augment that one with support from additional sources. There's evidence this turf war is breaking up, however. Recent polls have shown that medical doctors with conventional training are becoming far more open to alternative therapies like St. John's Wort, as are formerly conservative medical associations. For example, more than half of the MDs in the United States routinely prescribe some form of alternative therapy.

Still, the conventional therapies all have something going for them and shouldn't be eclipsed by the spotlight on St. John's Wort. Here's a look at what they can do for you.

What benefits can I get from conventional treatment?

That's an easy one: When effective, you can expect relief from some or all of depression's immediate symptoms within two months; you can also expect an end to a current episode of the disorder (called its acute phase) and a return to health (called remission) within three to four months. When effective, continued therapy also increases the chances of prevention of a relapse episode or any new episodes down the road; or in the case of bipolar disorder, a decrease or end to mood swings. Also, when one form of standard therapy is not helpful or, in the case of medication, has too many side effects, there is still a very good chance that another will work.

What kind of doctor should I see? What are my options?

The person making your diagnosis should be knowledgeable about the many treatment options available for psychiatric disorders. Most herbalists do not have this background, although a few have studied medicine. The more reputable herbalists will refer you to a practicing psychiatrist, psychologist, or other mental-health professional to obtain a diagnosis of your condition. A family physician might make that initial diagnosis.

If you know from the start that you want to treat your depression with alternative therapies, look for a medical professional who practices holistic healing, but has a thorough background in the diagnosis of mental disorders. It will probably be more difficult to find such a physician than it would be just to visit your local herbalist or homeopath, but is worth it in terms of increased opportunities for treatment. The most knowledgeable and sensitive of these physicians can combine the best of both worlds—conventional medicine's latest groundbreaking research on depression's sources and treatments with alternative medicine's noninvasive therapies. Look in the resource section for more information about how to find physicians who practice holistic medicine.

Here are the various types of caregivers you may encounter in your search for depression relief:

Primary Care Physician (PCP)—a physician with conventional medical training; practice addresses a wide range of mild to moderate illness; specialization in one field is not required. Usually, these physicians are board-eligible or certified in family practice or internal medicine. Although board certification does not ensure that a doctor is competent, it does increase the chances.

Psychiatrist—a medical doctor with at least three years advanced training in the assessment and treatment of mental disorders. As state-licensed MDs, psychiatrists are approved to dispense prescription drugs. Most psychiatrists also offer psychotherapy, although hour for hour these doctors are typically more expensive than other therapists.

Psychologist—someone with a broad base of knowledge in the psychological treatment of mental illness, as well as psychological causes and current theories; training usually involves a four-year postgraduate degree (including between two and four years' worth of part-time clinical training), followed by a one-year clinical internship. Clinical psychologists usually have a Ph.D. degree, although other doctoral degrees include Psy.D. and Ed.D. In some states, an experienced clinician with an M.A. or M.S. degree also may be licensed as a psychologist. Currently a point of controversy, psychologists are not permitted to prescribe medication.

Therapist—technically, anyone can call himself or herself a therapist, as the term is not tied to any governing body or accepted list of qualifications; this is a broad term often used to describe anyone who treats mental illness; unless a specific advanced degree in medicine, social work, or psychology is demonstrated, it could mean anything.

Counselor—again this is sometimes used as a broad term with no attendant qualifications; it usually describes someone with a degree from a one- or two-year postgraduate program.

Naturopath—a physician trained in conventional medicine who has also completed course work in nonconventional therapies such as acupuncture, botanical remedies, or therapeutic nutrition.

Homeopath—a health care worker who uses only plant-based therapies as treatments; he may or may not have any conventional medical training or be officially certified by recognized homeopathic organizations; in their training, most medical doctors learn, pejoratively, that a "homeopath" is a doctor who uses very small doses of medications that are unlikely to yield much more than a placebo response.

See Chapter Nine on organizations that can help you find reputable practitioners in your area.

What Those Initials Mean

You've seen them—the array of letters after your doctor's name above the doorbell. You've figured out MD (medical doctor), but what do the others mean?

- *MB or MBBS (Medical Baccalaureate or Medical Baccalaureate and Bachelor of Science)*—sometimes the equivalent of an MD degree, granted by programs in the United Kingdom and British Commonwealth.
- *DO (Doctor of Osteopathy)*—a physician trained at an osteopathic medical school. Although differences in MDs and DOs are decreasing, osteopathic training continues to include the "art" of manipulation of joints and bones.
- *Ph.D. (Doctor of Philosophy)*—the conventional degree for nonphysicians, this reflects postgraduate training that concentrated heavily on academic research and theory.
- *Psy.D. (Doctor of Psychology)*—an alternate professional degree in psychology that reflects a specialization in emotional, behavioral, and psychological disorders, without rigorous research training.
- *MSW (Masters in Social Work)*—a degree denoting completion of a program for those in social service, involving coursework, internships and practical experience; no clinical background is ensured.

continued

- *ACSW (Accredited Clinical Social Worker)*—this is the equivalent in having your "boards" in social work; all MSW's who are ACSW have bona fide clinical training.
- *MFCC (Master's in Family and Child Counseling)*— certification involves training in therapy techniques and counseling, with a focus on family dynamics.
- *CAC (Certified Addiction Counselor)*—a counselor who has completed one year of advanced study in addictive disorders.

How do I find a good doctor or therapist?

Ask around. Don't probe just anyone, however, but target your search among those whose opinions in this serious matter you value. Obviously, if you know someone already in therapy, that would be a good person to speak with. If you feel uncomfortable talking about your condition with coworkers, friends, or family, try to overcome that feeling; these are the very people who should be involved in your treatment, providing you with a support network. If you cannot discuss mental illness with this network, be creative about seeking other sources. When asking for information from people, you might phrase the question in a way that makes them think more carefully about their answers, like: "If someone you loved had depression, who do you trust enough to send them to for help?" Here are some sources you might tap for referrals:

- Doctors—your primary-care physician and any other doctor you typically see, such as a gynecologist, should be able to supply some names
- Professional associations (some are listed in the resource chapter)
- Depression support groups—check your local paper and community bulletin boards to see when these groups meet and try to talk to organizers and leaders
- Schools and universities—medical colleges and schools offering courses in conventional and alternative therapies may provide lists of reputable local practitioners
- Hospitals—these will sometimes recommend doctors af-

filiated with them; target hospitals noted for the quality of
their mental-health care

- Ads and referral services—take the information provided
  by these with a grain of salt; referral services are often
  paid by those they list—use these to find out the basics
  of background and specialty or if you have no other avenues of information
- Health-food stores—if alternative medicine is the only
  kind you'll consider, people who work in these shops may
  have heard customers' recommendations (again, however,
  beware)
- Phone hot lines—suicide hot lines and other nonprofit
  phone services may be able to refer you to qualified therapists
- Spiritual advisors—priests, rabbis, and other religious
  counselors may be able to direct you

**I want to shop around to get the best treatment. But I
haven't got a clue how to compare doctors. What should
I look for?**

Well, what *are* you looking for? Before you go shopping,
make sure you are clear in your own head about what it is
you want from a health-care provider. It's often helpful to talk
things over with a friend, who might be able to see a pattern
in what you're looking for and have insights into what personalities would work best with you.

When you go "shopping," take along a list—prepare questions you can use to screen doctors. Start with something very
basic and open-ended to initiate a revealing discussion, such
as "How would you go about determining a treatment for
me?" or "What if I don't understand something you've told
me?" If you don't like the direction the answer takes or are
frustrated with a dismissive, uninformative response, chances
are this is not a good match for you. Everyone is unique and
will want something different from the doctor/patient relationship. Some people want their doctor to take control, others
prefer the relationship to be more of a collaboration. Obviously, education, hospital affiliation, and experience will all
play roles in your decision, as will financial considerations.
But basically it should be about feeling comfortable. Do you
feel like you could openly discuss your condition with this

person? Do you believe he or she will give you honest, thorough answers to your questions? Does this person seem to really care about depression and its treatment? These are the things that will most likely guide you to the appropriate caregiver. Here are some more questions to get you started:

WHAT TO ASK DOCTORS

. . . *Before Your First Visit*

How much will the first visit cost and how can I pay for it?

Will I be required to pay for any tests on that first visit?

What kind of information will the doctor need?

How long does it take to get an appointment?

How long is a session?

. . . *About Their Training, Background, and Focus*

How long have you been in practice?

What is your background?

Are you licensed and board-certified?

In what areas do you specialize?

What interests you about the mood disorders?

What is your ''philosophy'' toward treatment?

What do you think causes depression?

How many patients do you see in a week who have a condition similar to mine?

What kind of success rate have you observed in people with this problem?

. . . *About How You Will Work Together*

What should I do about questions I may have between visits?

How do I schedule visits?

How often will we need to see each other?

What happens if I need to see another kind of specialist or want a second opinion?

What if there's some type of emergency?

. . . *About Your Condition*

What's wrong with me? What exactly is my diagnosis?

Why am I vulnerable to this condition?

Do you have any literature or can you recommend good
   sources of information on this condition?
What's my future going to be like with this?
Does my condition really require treatment?

... *About Your Therapy*

What are my treatment options?
What kind of response can I expect?
How will we decide what to try first?
When will we accept that something's not working?
What happens if several therapies are tried, but fail?
What will I need to do to make my treatment successful?
Are there organizations that can give me information and
   help?
Are support groups available?
How will I feel during the treatment? Afterward?
What are the pros and cons of this therapy?
How long will I be on this therapy?

... *About Tests*

What kinds of tests might I need?
What do they do?
Do I really need them?
How can I find out more about them?
What can I expect?
How much do they cost? Are they covered by insurance?
Who schedules them?
How often should I get each one?
When will you get the results? How will I find out what
   they are?
What do I need to do to prepare for this test?

... *About Prescription Drugs*

What is the name of the drug—its generic and brand
   names? (ask the doctor to write the name legibly if
   you have trouble with it)
Are there differences between brands?
Is there any literature on this that I can take away with
   me?
Why is this drug being chosen? What can it do for me?
How does it work?

What kind of change should I expect to notice? How soon?

How much should I take?

When should it be taken?

How long should it be taken?

Should it be taken with food?

Are there any interactions with food or other drugs I should be aware of?

What happens if I miss a dose?

Can I overdose on this drug?

What are the side effects?

If I'm pregnant or nursing, what risks does this have for my baby?

Is there a less-expensive, generic form that will offer me the same results?

Do I need to taper off gradually, or can I just stop using it?

If I do want to stop the therapy, will I need a "wash-out" period before I can try another drug?

. . . About Money Issues

How much is a typical visit?

What happens if I have to cancel an appointment? How much notice must I give? Will I have to pay?

What insurance plans are accepted?

What is the payment policy? Can you bill the insurance company directly or do I have to pay the fees "up-front"?

Do you have a sliding fee scale for people who aren't covered by insurance?

Will the doctor's office work with me if I need a payment plan?

How much will any tests cost?

What is the average cost for therapy for this condition?

Are there less-expensive treatment options that are successful addressing my problem?

What kinds of things will a doctor or therapist ask me?

If that list daunts you or you get flustered and are worried you won't give accurate responses, write answers out before you go, or, perhaps, Xerox or tear out these pages to take with you. Research your family medical history and take notes on it with you to the doctor's office. During an episode of depression, keep a record of your symptoms as you notice them, so you can be accurate and clear when describing them to your doctor. Ask friends and family members what symptoms they have observed. Try to remember what your response has been to other treatments in the past. Make notes on what your doctor is asking and the things she tells you—bring along a tape recorder if note-taking is not your forte. (Remember, you should ask permission to record a session. If your doctor balks at this, explain that your concentration is poor and this will cut down the need for follow-up phone calls!) And when you answer: Be honest! Don't hide things from doctors. If a caregiver makes negative value judgments—not clinical observations—about your response to depression, he or she may not be the right caregiver for you in this situation.

A thorough and reputable physician will cover these things in depth during your first interview:

- Current symptoms
- Past symptoms
- Any suicidal tendencies
- A detailed personal medical history, including conditions not apparently related to depression
- A detailed family medical history, focusing on psychiatric disorders but covering other health conditions that run in the family
- Current life situation—work, social relationships, family, social, school, spiritual
- Number of past pregnancies and typical pattern of menstrual cycles
- Medications you are currently taking; this will include any maintenance drugs such as birth control
- Prior treatments attempted—names and dosages of drugs, period of treatment, and level of compliance (how consistent you were in carrying out the treatment). Again: Tell the truth! This is the time to reveal any problems you have with carrying out a drug regimen, since those facts will influence the first-line therapy your doctor suggests

Your therapist might also ask to speak with family members or friends you feel would give an accurate, fair picture of your symptoms as viewed from the "outside." Although it is your right to refuse this, it's generally a good idea. By law, your therapist can only contact a family member, spouse, friend, etc., without your permission in an emergency or life-threatening circumstance.

What if I can't afford the doctor I want or the treatment I need?

First, don't assume there's no room for negotiation. Many therapists offer sliding fees to patients with inadequate medical insurance, basing their rates on what the client can afford to pay. Others will work with you to come up with a payment plan that makes treatment more viable. If you like your doctor, chances are that person is a caring individual who wants to see you get better and will work with you to make it happen.

Next, weigh the outlay against the long-term benefits. Are you losing money from lost work? Will absenteeism or poor productivity from untreated depression jeopardize your job and future income? It may be a struggle to pay for treatment now, but it could be cheaper for you in the end.

Finally, fight for what you want and need. Don't settle for a simple "no" from an insurance company. Pester them with regular calls—enlist friends and family if this is beyond you in your present state of depression. Talk with your employer about an Employee Assistance Plan (EAP) or with your welfare case manager. Find out about your county's mental health benefit program. Write firm letters outlining what's needed and ask your doctor's office to provide one saying the treatment is necessary in order to prevent future hospitalization and higher long-term medical bills. See if your doctor employs someone to deal with insurance companies; turn the whole issue over to that person, who has experience extracting money from reluctant providers. Keep in mind that a perceived roadblock is sometimes the mind's way of avoiding an unpleasant or shameful task—and there need be no shame in getting help for depression!

If there is, after all, no room for negotiation, work within the system. Ask for information and referrals to doctors covered by your insurance plan and ask your current physician to look over the list with you. Try to keep an open mind when meeting new doctors. You might find a therapist every bit as good as the one you initially wanted and treatment options that will work for you.

What is pharmacotherapy?

Simply put, it is the use of medication to treat a medical illness or disorder. In terms of depression, pharmacotherapy is the best-studied and documented of the therapy options for depression, as well as for the prevention of repeated episodes or relapse. Antidepressant drugs are often the first line of treatment for the more severe cases of mental illness. Medications are often used in conjunction with psychotherapy.

Can drugs cure depression?

The term "cure" is usually used to convey that a person has not only recovered from an illness fully, but also that the illness process has been totally eliminated or rectified. For example, an appendectomy is the "cure" for acute appendicitis. From this perspective, there is no cure for depression. Because the disorder is not a disease, but a collection of symptoms resulting from complex, multidetermined causes, it is difficult to target a true "cure." What drugs can do is dampen the impact of depression symptoms and, over four to six weeks, temporarily repair a biochemical malfunction connected to the disorder. That's no small potatoes. By alleviating symptoms, antidepressants allow people with mood disturbances to function and gives them the breathing space they need to work on solving the problems associated with depression pain. When people are placed on a type of drug therapy appropriate to their mood disorders and follow it to the letter, they can expect about a 60% chance of success in treating the condition. If pharmacotherapy is given three or four chances, response rates of 80 to 90% can be expected.

If antidepressant drugs are so great, why do they have a bad reputation?

It's clear they do suffer from a PR problem. Despite the fact that they have been demonstrated time and time again as effective and safe in the treatment of depression, a Gallup poll conducted in 1993 revealed that 25 percent of people polled would refuse to use antidepressants.

There are a number of factors behind this unpopularity. Some people are reluctant to use any form of drug therapy, period, even aspirin. Others have had bad experiences with a drug—anything from an antibiotic to a pain reliever. Some berate antidepressants as treating only the symptoms of mood disorder; the drugs may be alleviating the pain, but they are not addressing and eliminating underlying psychological and emotional stressors. But much of the antidrug sentiment arises from the fact that high numbers of people treated with drugs for their symptoms were simply never given the correct medications for mood disorder, or did not give an appropriate treatment a legitimate trial—maybe they stopped taking it before it had time to work or were using it in combination with other therapies that interfered with its actions. Failure of the medication to bring relief raised a barrier to drugs as a whole. Fear of potential side effects is another barrier. For some, the idea of medications that alter brain chemistry conjures up images of "big brother," mind control, or zombie-like indifference. Finally, social stigma is involved. Therapeutic medications are sometimes lumped together with drugs of abuse or "recreational" misuse. Somehow, taking medication is perceived as an acknowledgment of weakness. Oddly, considering it is labeled "alternative," I've found many people much more open to self-medication with an herbal tea than to accepting the idea they might need a drug to cope.

Do drugs work on every kind of mood disorder?

Certain types of medication have been shown to be effective for every type of mood disorder, but their effects on milder forms of depression are not too much greater than that of placebos—in other words, in studies of drug effects, people with very mild episodes of depression were almost as likely to feel better from doses of what they simply believed to be a prescription drug (but which was actually a nonreactive pretender) as they were from true drug therapies. Does this mean the depression was "all in their head"? Yes or no, depending on what you mean. It may be that the chemical effects of mild depression are too subtle for observation or are impacting on some biochemical processes that aren't touched by these types of medications. Certainly, these results lend support to the theory that St. John's Wort is a viable alternative for the treatment of milder types of mood disorder. It is also true that people with milder acute symptoms are typically less impaired at work or home and have more normal sleep and hormonal profiles. For these people, the support of others, the prospects of receiving professional help, and the passage of time have powerful healing or recuperative effects.

Psychotic mood disorders, whether "just" depression or bipolar disorder, do not respond as well to use of a single drug therapy as more moderate cases. But these extreme cases also do not respond well to placebo. Alternative herbal remedies have shown negligible results on these severe cases. For these, a combination of drug treatments involving an antidepressant and an antipsychotic or (for bipolar illness) a mood stabilizer, or a combination of drug and electroconvulsive therapy seems called for. Herbalists, counselors, and homeopaths have no place in treating these illnesses *unless* in collaboration with a qualified psychiatrist.

So, what overall effects should I expect from my drug therapy?

Don't expect a sudden rush of euphoria from an antidepressant. First of all, most antidepressants must be taken for at least several weeks before any effect is felt, but also, these drugs don't produce sensations of happiness or high energy; they simply alleviate feelings of sadness and worry. What you *should* notice is a gradual lifting of the gray curtain of depression—the dulling effect of persistent low mood. Improvements in sleep, libido, sense of humor and concentration should follow over the next several weeks. While the result may be dramatic in terms of the sense of release, it's nothing as theatrical as cocaine's high.

Expect some mild side effects—these are medications after all, and they are being taken on a regular basis. Side effects will vary according to the drug being used. You'll reduce the chances of these if you follow dosing instructions carefully and if you and your doctor work from the ground up—that is, start with the lowest dose that seems appropriate and move up to higher ones if needed. Then, expect to see some benefit.

This will not happen overnight. Just as St. John's Wort may take up to six weeks to show its effects, a drug therapy needs to build up in your system for its full action to be noted. Talk to your doctor about how long you should wait before looking for relief.

If you and your doctor work diligently together and, if necessary, you're willing to go through a trial and error sequence of three or four medications, you'll have an 80 to 90 percent chance of responding well to antidepressants. If you stay on the therapy for the full course of the continuation phase (a minimum of six months after the episode ends), you shouldn't expect a relapse. Risk of relapse plunges from an untreated high of 60 percent to just 10 to 20 percent if you remain on continuation therapy. After the six-month period is up, expect a full recovery. If not, changes in the treatment plan can be made. Even people with a history of repeated episodes can expect a sustained recovery if they remain on maintenance treatment over the next few years.

I finally saw my doctor for my depression and anxiety, but when my doctor talked about the ways that we could treat it, I was totally confused. The doctor said we could use either "tricyclics, SSRIs, or perhaps an MAOI." I had no idea what he was talking about, but I was too embarrassed to ask any questions.

There's no reason to feel foolish if you don't know anything about the drugs that your doctor says might work well for treating your depression and anxiety. There are a very large number of medications that can be used for these conditions. If your doctor won't or can't take the time to explain these drugs to you, you might think about finding another who will treat you more like a partner.

The following is a short summary of the main types of drugs that can be used to treat depression and anxiety: tricyclic antidepressants (tricyclics, TCAs), selective serotonin re-uptake inhibitors (SSRIs), monoamine oxidase inhibitors (MAOIs), and the so-called atypical antidepressants. All of these drugs work by changing the activity of specific chemicals in the brain that may be at abnormal levels in people with depression. Some other drugs that might be used along with these antidepressants are also reviewed.

TRICYCLIC ANTIDEPRESSANTS

This group of drugs has been around for almost forty years and has a large number of members that are listed immediately below. The drugs are called tricyclics because their chemical structures have three rings.

Class members

This class includes Anafranil (clomipramine hydrochloride), Aventyl or Pamelor (nortriptyline hydrochloride), Elavil (amitriptyline hydrochloride), Norpramin or Pertofrane (desipramine hydrochloride), Sinequan or Adapin (doxepin hydrochloride), Surmontil (trimipramine maleate), Tofranil or Janimine (imipramine hydrochloride), Triavil (a combination of amitriptyline and perphanazine), and Vivactil (protriptyline hydrochloride).

How they work

All TCAs are thought to work by raising the ability of selected chemicals in the brain to influence nerve cells. These drugs prevent nerve cells that release two important brain chemicals (neurotransmitters), norepinephrine and serotonin, from taking them back up after the cells "fire" or send their signals. Preventing this makes norepinephrine and serotonin work at closer to normal levels and thus relieves depression.

Restoring levels of norepinephrine or serotonin are probably just the first step of a series of neurochemical reactions. The tricyclic affects the "inner life" of both the cell that sends the signal (called the pre-synaptic neuron) and the cell that receives the signal (called the post-synaptic neuron). Changes inside these cells influence the ability to receive further signals (by increasing or decreasing the number of neurotransmitter "receivers" or receptors) and the activity of various genes. It probably takes at least three to four weeks for an antidepressant to cause all of these changes within nerve cells.

Not all TCAs work in exactly the same way. Some drugs (nortriptyline, protriptyline, and desipramine) have much greater effects on norepinephrine than serotonin, while the others raise the effects of both of these neurotransmitters. We used to think that Elavil and Anafranil were more selective for serotonin, but because both of these drugs have powerful metabolites that affect norepinephrine, it's now clear that they are not selective.

Potential problems

Almost any drug that you take for any illness has potential side effects and TCAs are no exception to this rule. Many of the side effects that occur with TCAs result from the fact that they can influence a variety of other chemical systems in the brain and other parts of the body in addition to norepinephrine and serotonin.

Common side effects of TCAs include constipation, sedation, dry mouth, dizziness, and weight gain. All of these tend to occur more often with the drugs that affect both norepinephrine and serotonin than with those that primarily affect norepinephrine. Tricyclics can also produce fainting spells by causing decreases in blood pressure when changing postures, especially in older patients and those with heart problems. Other side effects that may occur during treatment with a TCA include fatigue, nausea, vomiting, headache, hallucinations, rapid and/or irregular heartbeat, confusion, and decreased desire for sex (libido). While the list of *potential* side effects for TCAs is long, it is important to remember that chances of experiencing any one of them is small. This is also true for all of the other drugs considered in this chapter.

You have to be careful when taking TCAs because it is possible for an overdose to be lethal. As little as a seven- to ten-day supply of these drugs can be fatal if all the pills are taken at once. Also, be doubly careful to prevent children from accidentally taking these medications.

Like all drugs, the body processes TCAs to remove them. For most TCAs, this involves chemical reactions in the liver. Many other drugs that might be used to treat heart problems and other conditions are processed in a similar way. Thus, when you are taking a TCA and another drug, levels of one or both in your body may become too high or low. It is very important that your doctor knows all the other drugs you are taking when he prescribes a TCA for you.

While TCAs can be associated with unpleasant side effects

and are very dangerous when mistakenly taken in very large doses, they have been used safely in a very large number of patients for a very long time.

Why should I take a TCA?

While there are many newer drugs for treating depression, TCAs are still prescribed very often for this condition. There are good reasons for this. First, these drugs may work in as many as 40–60% of people whose depression is not relieved by newer drugs that are discussed below. Second, many TCAs are available as generics (like ibuprofen for Advil) and are thus relatively inexpensive. Third, many of the drugs in this class work well for the treatment of depression and other conditions that may often occur along with it including anxiety or chronic pain.

Important points about particular TCAs

Anafranil—Treatment with this TCA can produce all of the side effects mentioned above and it may also increase sensitivity of the skin to sunlight (i.e., how easily you sunburn). Thus, if you are taking this TCA, you should avoid excessive sunlight. This same problem can occur if you are taking either Tofranil (Janimine) or Vivactil. Anafranil should not be taken in doses higher than 250 mg/day to avoid a higher risk of seizures. Anafranil is used throughout the world to treat depression, although in the U.S. it is only approved for the treatment of obsessive-compulsive disorder.

Elavil, Sinequan, and Tofranil—These TCAs should be avoided if you have a history of heart disease or glaucoma. Older people tend to have a harder time taking these medications (constipation, blurry vision, urinary retention).

Norpramin and Pamelor—These medications may not work as well when the dose is too high. It should always be prescribed in the smallest dose that relieves symptoms because taking very large amounts of the drug can be fatal. Some doctors prefer them for treatment of older patients because they tend to have fewer side effects.

Triavil—In addition to the side effects noted above, treatment with this combination medication for several years or longer can result in difficulties in making simple everyday movements (doctors refer to this problem as "tardive dyskinesia"). Triavil probably should only be used for treatment of psychotic depression.

SELECTIVE SEROTONIN RE-UPTAKE INHIBITORS

This group of antidepressant drugs is much newer than TCAs and is now the class used most often for the treatment of depression in the United States.

Class members

This class includes *Prozac* (fluoxetine hydrochloride), *Zoloft* (sertraline hydrochloride), *Paxil* (paroxetine hydrochloride), and *Luvox* (fluvoxamine maleate).

How they work

All SSRIs work in the same way. As their name would suggest, SSRIs (also called serotonin uptake blockers) reduce the ability of brain cells that release serotonin to take it back up. It is this effect of SSRIs that is generally thought to make them effective for relieving depression. This action is shared by many of the TCAs discussed above. However, SSRIs are much more specific in their actions than TCAs. They have little or no influence on other brain chemicals, including norepinephrine. This specificity is also the reason why SSRIs have fewer and less serious side effects than TCAs.

Selective serotonin re-uptake inhibitors are useful for treating a wide range of psychiatric conditions in addition to depression, including anxiety, panic attacks, and obsessive-compulsive disorder.

Potential problems

While SSRIs have been repeatedly shown to cause fewer side effects than TCAs and to be much less dangerous in overdose, you may experience some problems when taking them. Side effects of SSRIs include headache, insomnia, and feelings of restlessness or nervousness. Selective serotonin re-uptake

inhibitors may also cause sexual side effects, particularly de-
layed orgasm. If you have a history of seizures, heart disease,
or extreme excitement (mania), SSRIs should be taken with
caution.

Selective serotonin re-uptake inhibitors, like TCAs, are
processed in the liver for removal from the body. As you
would expect from what was noted above for TCAs, taking
SSRIs along with other drugs may result in levels in the body
that are too high or low. Here again, it is very important that
your doctor knows all the other drugs you are taking because
that may make a difference in the SSRI that your doctor prescribes for you.

Selective serotonin re-uptake inhibitors should never be
taken with an MAOI and several weeks without treatment
should be permitted to occur if you and your doctor decide to
switch from one class to the other. The presence of an SSRI
and an MAOI in your body at the same time may result in an
adverse event referred to as "serotonin syndrome."

Abruptly stopping treatment or missing doses of an SSRI
may result in gastrointestinal complaints, flu-like symptoms,
sleep disturbance, and psychological symptoms including anxiety and irritability. The chances of experiencing these problems when stopping treatment with an SSRI can be reduced
by slowly decreasing the dose over a period of weeks (taper-
ing). In any case, these symptoms tend to be short-lived and
relatively mild. It should also be mentioned that the ability of
SSRIs to relieve the most severe depression has not been well
studied. Nevertheless, they are widely considered as the first
choice for management of mild to moderately severe depression.

Why should I take an SSRI?

Selective serotonin re-uptake inhibitors are generally safer
and easier to take than TCAs. Selective serotonin re-uptake
inhibitors have been studied extensively in a wide range of
individuals with depression and been shown to be as effective
as, and better tolerated than, TCAs. As noted above, SSRIs
are generally considered as the first choice for treatment of
mild to moderately severe depression.

Since they are relatively new, SSRIs are not available as
generics (in the U.S., this will occur for the first member of

this class, Prozac, in 2002). Thus, using an SSRI to treat your depression will probably be more expensive than a TCA in the short run.

Treatment with an SSRI should be started with the lowest dose that might be expected to relieve depression. This will reduce cost and minimize the possibility of side effects.

A final point to remember regarding SSRIs is that the drugs in this class are similar in how well they work in treating depression as well as their side effects. The SSRI that your doctor prescribes for you may depend largely on his or her personal experience and preferences as well as other medication that you may be taking. However, Luvox is only approved in the U.S. for treatment of obsessive-compulsive disorder.

Important points about particular SSRIs

Prozac—It is the SSRI first used widely to treat depression. It remains in the body for a very long time after treatment is stopped and particular care must be taken with switching from Prozac to another antidepressant medication, particularly an MAOI.

Paxil—This SSRI may be more likely than other drugs in the class to interact with other medications you may be taking. Make particularly sure your doctor knows about all of your medications if you are going to start therapy with Paxil. Withdrawal symptoms may occur more often with Paxil than with Prozac.

Zoloft—Although the average dose of Zoloft prescribed by psychiatrists is between 100-150 mg per day, it can be effective in as little as 50 mg daily doses. If you respond to this lower dose, there is less chance for medication interactions and you can save money by taking one-half of a 100 mg tablet. The same also may be true for Paxil at 10 mg per day.

MONOAMINE OXIDASE INHIBITORS

This class of drugs has been used to treat depression for many years. They work well in many patients, but they may require more careful use than either TCAs or SSRIs.

Class members

This class includes *Nardil* (phenelzine sulfate) and *Parnate* (tranylcypromine sulfate).

How they work

Monoamine oxidase inhibitors are older drugs, like the TCAs. The MAOIs raise levels of serotonin, norepinephrine, and another chemical, dopamine, in the brain, but they do it in a completely different way than either TCAs or SSRIs. Monoamine oxidase inhibitors stop the normal breakdown of these neurotransmitters. The increased brain level of serotonin or norepinephrine that results from MAOI treatment is thought to be the main reason why these drugs work to relieve depression.

Potential problems

In addition to raising brain levels of serotonin, norepinephrine, and dopamine, MAOIs also increase the amounts of some other chemicals in your body, including the amino acid tyramine. If the amount of tyramine in your body, becomes too high, it can result in increased blood pressure (hypertension) and even in a condition referred to as a "hypertensive crisis."

There are a large number of foods that contain relatively high amounts of tyramine and these should be avoided if your depression is being treated with an MAOI. These foods include:

- Aged cheeses
- Preserved or smoked meats (e.g., summer sausage, or pre-packaged lunch meats)
- Pickled or smoked fish
- Some beans (Italian broad beans or fava beans)
- Yeast extracts
- Sauerkraut
- Large amounts of chocolate or caffeine
- Dried or over-ripe fruits
- Red wine, beer, and "colored" spirits (e.g., bourbon or scotch)

If your lifestyle does not permit you to closely monitor your diet, an MAOI should probably not be chosen to treat your depression.

Monoamine oxidase inhibitors may change levels of a wide range of other drugs in your body, including most over-the-counter cold and flu remedies, diet pills, stimulants, cocaine, and many other antidepressants. These drugs can also cause hypertensive crises and the serotonin syndrome.

Side effects that may occur during treatment with an MAOI include sudden drops in blood pressure upon standing (orthostatic hypotension), seizures, headache, and upset stomach, weight gain, sedation, insomnia, and low libido. These drugs may also make you more susceptible to sunburn.

If you have a history of diabetes, asthma, or low blood pressure, you should avoid taking an MAOI.

Why should I take an MAOI?

Monoamine oxidase inhibitors can work to relieve depression and anxiety when other types of drugs have failed. These drugs also work well in patients with atypical depression. I consider these antidepressants to be a third- or fourth-line choice for most patients.

HETEROCYCLIC ("TRICYCLIC-LIKE") AND NOVEL ANTIDEPRESSANTS

Heterocyclic antidepressants are relatively new drugs that may be used to relieve depression that has failed to respond to other drugs including TCAs and SSRIs.

Class members

Heterocyclic antidepressants include *Ascendin* (amoxapime), *Ludiomil* (maprotiline hydrochloride), *Serzone* (nefazodone hydrochloride), *Desyrel* (trazodone hydrochloride), and *Effexor* (venlafaxine). The tetracyclic antidepressant *Remeron* (mirtazapine) might also be considered together with these drugs.

How they work

We generally know less about these antidepressants than the other drugs discussed above. However, it appears that their primary effects also are on serotonin and norepinephrine. It appears that they interfere with the re-uptake of these chemicals in a way similar to the TCAs and SSRIs and that they also block the actions of this brain chemical on some of the cells that it normally influences. Some of the drugs in this class may also interfere with the uptake of norepinephrine by the cells which release it. Remeron appears to differ from other agents in this group in that it blocks serotonin from acting on specific groups of cells in the brain and enhances norepinephrine and serotonin without blocking their reuptake.

Potential problems

Heterocyclic antidepressants are less likely to cause serious side effects than TCAs, but you may still experience some problems when taking them for treatment of depression. Side effects of heterocyclic antidepressants include muscle and joint pain, upset stomach, drowsiness, and blurred vision. If you have a medical history that includes heart or liver disease you should use drugs in this class with caution. People with seizure disorders should not take Ludiomil. Desyrel has been reported to (rarely) cause prolonged and painful erections. Serzone should not be taken with certain prescription antihistimines. Higher doses of Effexor may cause increased blood pressure. Like Triavil, Asendin can cause tardive dyskinesia.

Why should I take a heterocyclic antidepressant?

These drugs do not appear to work better in relieving depression than the agents such as TCAs. However, they are much less likely than tricyclics to cause serious side effects.

The heterocyclic antidepressants are relatively new drugs and most will not be available as generics for some time. Thus, the cost of treating your depression with a heterocyclic drug is likely to be higher than therapy with an older drug such as a TCA. Desyrel is widely available as generic trazodone and it is commonly used in lower doses as a sleeping pill.

AMINOKETONE ANTIDEPRESSANTS

Wellbutrin (bupropion hydrochloride) is the only aminoketone approved for the treatment of depression. How this drug affects the brain to relieve depression is not well understood. It appears to block the re-uptake of dopamine by the cells which release it, and it has an enhancing effect on norepinephrine in the brain. Wellbutrin does not have a direct effect on serotonin.

Like other recently developed drugs used to treat depression, Wellbutrin is less likely to cause serious side effects than TCAs. Side effects of Wellbutrin include constipation, dry mouth, dizziness, headache, insomnia, upset stomach, and blurred vision. It may also cause a slight weight loss. In high doses, Wellbutrin can increase the risk of seizures.

Wellbutrin appears to be as effective as either TCAs, SSRIs, or heterocyclic drugs in relieving symptoms of depression. A second form of Wellbutrin, called Zyban, has been approved to help people stop smoking.

BENZODIAZEPINES

Benzodiazepines are a very large class of drugs that are often used to relieve anxiety. They are not antidepressants in the same sense as TCAs, SSRIs, MAOIs, or atypical drugs.

Class members

Drugs in this class are generally referred to as tranquilizers, but also include sleeping pills. The most commonly prescribed benzodiazepines include *Ativan* (lorazepam), *Centrax* (prazepram), *Dalmane* (flurazepam hydrochloride), *Halcion* (triazolam), *Klonopin* (clonazepam), *Librium* (chlordiazepoxide), *Limbitrol* (chlordiazepoxide plus amitriptyline hydrochloride), *Restoril* (temazepam), *Tranxene* (chlorazepate dipotassium), *Valium* (diazepam), and *Xanax* (alprazolam).

How they work

Benzodiazepines are thought to decrease anxiety by increasing the effectiveness of a specific brain chemical that quiets nerve cells, gamma aminobutyric acid (GABA). Benzodiazepines appear to have their greatest effect in parts of the brain that control emotional behavior. Benzodiazepines also effect brain levels of serotonin, norepinephrine, and dopamine.

Potential problems

Benzodiazepines may be given by mistake when chronic mild depression (dysthymia) is misdiagnosed as a "neurotic" condition. Side effects that you may experience during treatment with a benzodiazepine include movement problems, memory impairment, dizziness, sedation, confusion, orthostatic hypotension, and drowsiness. This last side effect makes sense since some of the drugs in this class (e.g., Dalmane, Halcion, Restoril) are used as sleeping pills. Although not too dangerous in overdose by themselves, the benzodiazepines will greatly strengthen the dangerousness of alcohol or other sedatives.

Benzodiazepines are processed for removal from the body in the liver and, like TCAs and SSRIs, they may interact with many other drugs.

Long term treatment with benzodiazepines may also result in the body developing a "need" for these drugs (physiologic dependence) and fairly intense discomfort if one abruptly stops taking them. Abrupt withdrawal after longer term treatment can cause seizures.

If you have a medical history that includes glaucoma, kidney or liver disease, suicidal tendencies, or drug or alcohol abuse, you should avoid taking most benzodiazepines. You should also avoid alcohol if you are taking a benzodiazepine.

Why should I take a benzodiazepine?

If you are highly anxious or your symptoms include panic, your doctor may prescribe a benzodiazepine. These drugs are very effective in providing short-term relief from anxiety and panic disorders and anxiety associated with depression.

MISCELLANEOUS AGENTS USED IN THE
TREATMENT OF DEPRESSION

Your doctor may suggest one or more drugs in addition to those mentioned above to treat your depression.

If you have a bipolar disorder, your doctor may suggest a mood stabilizer in addition to an antidepressant. Lithium carbonate (lithium salt) can even out mood swings in both directions. It generally works well in returning mood to normal levels and can increase the positive effect of your antidepressant medication. Side effects that may occur with lithium include upset stomach, drowsiness, weakness, dry mouth, tremors, increased thirst, and frequent urination. High doses of lithium can have toxic effects. If you have a medical history that includes thyroid, kidney or heart disease, or epilepsy, lithium should be used with caution.

Depakote (divalproex sodium)—Most commonly used for the treatment of seizures, but it can also be employed to treat mania and to prevent relapse of bipolar disorder. Side effects that may occur with Depakote include depression of brain activity, liver failure, problems in blood clotting, rash, and stomach upset. Depakote should be used with caution if you have a history of liver problems. Another anti-seizure drug, carbamazapine, also is used to treat manic depression.

Ritalin (methylphenidate hydrochloride)—Not an antidepressant. It is a mild brain stimulant that works to control hyperactivity, impulsiveness, and inattention that occurs with attention-deficit hyperactivity disorder (ADHD). By easing the symptoms of ADHD, Ritalin can help boost self-esteem and reduce mild associated depression. Side effects that may occur with Ritalin include sleep disturbances, nervousness, changes in blood pressure, dizziness, drowsiness, fever, and stomach upset. Ritalin can be abused for its stimulant effects and can become habit-forming. If your medical history includes glaucoma, high blood pressure, epilepsy or drug or alcohol abuse, Ritalin should be taken with caution.

Buspar (buspirone)—This is a nonaddictive anti-anxiety medication that works, indirectly, by strengthening one type of serotonin effect in the brain. Buspar is not rapidly effective, like a benzodiazepine, and must be taken on a daily basis.

Buspar is also used to enhance response to antidepressants and may reverse some SSRI side effects.

Which drug should I choose?

You shouldn't be making that decision alone! Obviously, your doctor will have a lot to say in the decision of which drug to use as a first line of therapy. Some doctors will not think to involve you in this decision at all—they will simply write out a prescription and hand it to you—unless you take matters into your own hands by asking questions.

All of the antidepressants currently on the market have about the same rate of success, and a similar time frame for their effects. Your doctor will typically consider your past history of treatment, the likelihood of particular side effects given your overall health, reaction to other medications you've taken in the past, and any allergic reactions you may have. The specific symptoms of depression you're experiencing will come into play as well—for instance, if you are having trouble with insomnia, tricyclics with sedating qualities, such as Serzone or Remeron, might be a first choice. If you admit to being irregular in your dosing, that factor will be taken into account. If you are suicidal, the doctor will probably avoid medications with a danger of toxic overdose. Cost may be an issue, too.

Don't be surprised if the first drug chosen is from the category of SSRIs. Those are currently the most popular first-choice medications. Their side effects tend to be less annoying and dosing easier than for other drugs. There is little chance of dying from an overdose on this type of antidepressant. SSRIs might not be prescribed if cost is a real issue, though. These are newer drugs, and so are still under patent. You can only buy them as brand-name medications, because generic versions are not yet available. If you require a higher dose of SSRIs, this can translate into an average of $120 to $150 more per month, much more than for older medications like tricyclics. But, before you cross SSRIs off the list consider this more-involved math: While in the short term, tricyclics and other older therapies available in generic form seem like the better therapeutic bargain, those older drugs tend to have harsher side effects, which in turn may necessitate more frequent doctor visits, the use of other medications to alleviate side effects, or laboratory tests. In six months, costs may even out or even tip the balance toward SSRIs when you take these costs into consideration.

I really don't like the idea of taking drugs or even St. John's Wort forever. I'd feel like an addict.

Do you consider diabetics who take insulin to treat their disease "addicts"? How about someone who takes Inderal for high blood pressure or Zantac for an ulcer? No one calls a patient receiving dialysis for kidney disease an "addict." Depression is an illness, just like those conditions, and drug therapy is one method doctors use to treat it.

It's true, though, that drug therapy for complete remission of depression requires a commitment over time. Here's what the research shows: A return to normal after an episode of depression is not the sign to stop drug treatment. The disorder is still "lurking," ready to swamp you at the least sign of vulnerability. If you discontinue your treatment immediately after the acute episode ends or even any time before six months of remission have passed, chances are at least fifty-fifty that you will slide back into the same episode. If you ride out the six-month "continuation phase" of the drug therapy, your chances of a relapse are much lower, although there is still the risk of later recurrence. During this period you would typically reduce the number of visits to a doctor from once a week to every two weeks or just once a month. If this is a first episode of the disorder—in other words a pattern of depression has not yet been established—then drug therapy is typically ended after this continuation phase is completed.

If, however, you've had a diagnosis of recurrent depression (you've had repeated attacks through the years) your doctor will probably recommend that you remain on drug maintenance for a while. Typically, maintenance therapy is taken for three or more years after the recurrent episode. Visits during this "maintenance phase" typically range from monthly to quarterly checkups. Maintenance will decrease your risk of repeated attacks to about 10 percent per year. Studies with placebos have shown this is a real effect of the drugs and not just a belief that they keep the symptoms at bay. Adding psychotherapy to drug therapy during this maintenance period may not significantly change recurrence figures, but can result in better coping strategies for relationships affected by the disorder. If the notion of drug treatment over a period of years makes you uncomfortable, some recent evidence suggests that cognitive behavior therapy or interpersonal psychotherapy can reduce the risk of depression after medication withdrawal. I *do not* recommend intermittent or "on again-off again" dosing because it might actually increase the frequency of relapsing episodes.

Why might treatment with medications be unsuccessful?

A variety of things could be responsible for unsuccessful treatment. Some can be traced to your doctor's role in the therapy: Was the drug really an appropriate choice for the disorder and its symptoms? Was the dose right? Or the duration long enough? How did it interact with other medications the patient was using? Did the doctor educate the patient in exactly how to take the medication and what contraindications to avoid? Did the physician provide all the information the patient and pharmacist needed?

Then again, the patient could be at fault: Was the medication taken as directed? How many doses were missed? Did the patient had a negative approach to the whole treatment, which could affect perception of its effectiveness? Did the patient have unreal expectations?

Or, it could be the result of factors beyond either person's control: The depression does not involve the brain systems influenced by this particular medication. Or side effects generate a nuisance factor that prevents you from dosing properly. Cost of therapy was prohibitive.

Finally, the patient might have been misdiagnosed. People who suffer from chronic depression, also known as dysthymia, are frequently treated for neurotic conditions instead of the mild depression they actually have. Once given the correct drug therapy, these people often experience a dramatic return to health. For years, they have simply been on the wrong medications.

What if a drug doesn't work?

If there was good reason to choose it and it has been well tolerated, try a larger dose. Doctors should always start patients on the low end of the dose spectrum and work up only if needed. Ask your doctor if you should try increasing your dose. Try again. If that doesn't work, shift to another medication from a different category. If that's a failure, maybe still another class of antidepressant will work.

Sometimes two drugs will be used in combination, like a TCA or MAOI and lithium. Drug therapy is sometimes augmented by thyroid hormones, the beta-blocker pindolol, or psychostimulants. Some doctors are mixing TCAs and SSRIs but data on the effects and safety of this polypharmacy, or multi-drug strategy, are still weak. If your doctor suggests this, ask why and if you should be alert to side effects.

However, a variety of factors will be involved in your decision on what to try next. If you are resistant enough to the idea of pharmacotherapy for your feelings to color your whole approach to drug treatment, discuss nonchemical options with your doctor.

Are antidepressants addictive?

True antidepressant therapies (as opposed to those sedatives sometimes mistakenly used to treat chronic depression) are typically not addictive. Their effect is to relieve depression's troubling symptoms by stabilizing distorted systems in the brain (i.e., to correct, or over-correct an abnormality). They do not generate pleasurable sensations that don't exist without the drug. They don't give you a "high" that you will begin to crave. For instance, if a nondepressive person were to take an antidepressant, no change in mood would be observed, only some side effects.

Who should be careful with drug therapy?

Everyone should be reasonably cautious taking an antidepressant—or for that matter, St. John's Wort or seeing a therapist. But you should also be cautiously optimistic that treatment will be helpful. Anyone experiencing overall ill health should be especially cautious when introducing a drug therapy and aware of potential side effects that could exacerbate existing problems. But there are also what doctors call "special populations" that should use special care:

Elderly patients—Effects of depression drug therapies may be more extreme in elderly patients, even those who are otherwise healthy. Lower doses or less frequent applications are usually indicated. Older people are more likely to be on a continuous regimen of medications, so the drug therapy should be considered in the bigger picture of possible drug-drug interactions. Elderly patients with memory problems are more likely to miss doses or accidentally overdose, so they should be monitored; drugs with less risk for overdose poisoning are better choices for these patients.

Pregnant or nursing women—Most drugs have not been studied for their effects on infants or increased risk for birth defects, and so should be avoided if a woman is planning to or has become pregnant. Psychotherapy may be the safer option here if the depression is not too severe. Trace amounts of medications make it into breast milk, so drugs should be avoided by nursing mothers as well.

Children—Young people can't be expected to be as responsible about drug therapy as adults, so the responsibility for monitoring them rests on a team of family members, caregivers, teachers, school nurses, and doctors. They'll need to keep an eye on dosing and be alert for side effects. Since children often won't volunteer this information, gentle prods will be necessary. And some kids will only pretend to take their medicine—make sure it's really going down. Children with mood disorders are prescribed many of the same therapies as adults, though in smaller doses. Kids with depression and attention deficit disorders present another challenge and should use stimulants only under careful supervision.

Drugs just aren't helping my depression. Should I switch to psychotherapy?

If it interests you, and your disorder doesn't rule it out, you should certainly try psychotherapy. But don't get your hopes up too high. Successful treatment with psychotherapy after a nonresponse to drugs is typically low—in one study just 30 percent found relief when they switched. Perhaps you could explore a combination of the two, or ask your doctor about considering medication from other categories of antidepressants. More options may exist now than when you first began your treatment.

What kinds of psychotherapy are used to treat depression?

There are a number of forms of psychotherapy commonly applied to depression and its symptoms. Clearly, these do not directly target any possible chemical causes for the disorder, but might indirectly have an impact even on those—for instance, breathing techniques that alter carbon dioxide levels and blood flow certainly can have chemical implications.

Here are a list of the therapies you are more likely to encounter; talk to your medical doctor about how they should fit into your treatment plan:

Interpersonal psychotherapy (IPT)—This is one of the newer forms of psychotherapy. It does not usually follow the more prolonged course common to analytic therapy, but instead is usually completed in just 3 or 4 months of weekly sessions. The therapist and patient use that time to help the depressed person develop better ways to handle stressful social interactions. In some recent studies, IPT was tested for effectiveness in the battle against recurrent depression—repeated episodes of major depression. It had a success rate of about one-third in those trials, a number which falls somewhere between those receiving treatment with antidepressants and those on placebo (people who thought they were receiving a medication but were actually being given nonactive fillers). In several studies, IPT was significantly less effective for patients who had very specific forms of sleep malfunction—decreased "delta" waves during the first period of deep sleep or increased Rapid Eye Movement (REM or dream) sleep. This may indicate that there is a level of brain disturbance in some depressions that basically "requires" medication treatment.

Behavioral Therapy—This form of therapy targets actions that have an impact on depression or anxiety symptoms. Typically, depressed people are helped to increase involvement in rewarding activities and to practice ways of coping with low moods. One therapy utilizes breathing exercises called "diaphragmatic breathing" which reduce sensations of anxiety. It is most successful when used to treat milder forms and episodes of depression. "Exposure therapy" provides guided experience in situations that provoke stress, anxiety, and mood disturbances in order to overcome avoidance or fearful behavior.

Cognitive-Behavioral Therapy (CBT)—This treatment addresses the negative feelings about self, world, and future so typical of depression, in the belief that these feelings of low self-esteem actually cause the symptoms of depression. Its techniques are designed to improve social interaction, shift focus away from depressive symptoms, and break the self-fulfilling prophecy of negative thinking. Patients learn coping strategies that prevent unhealthy reactions to stressors and to anxiety disorder symptoms. Like IPT, CBT may be more helpful for depressed people who aren't affected by too many disturbances of brain function. One could make a case that IPT or CBT would be good "standards" against which to measure the effectiveness of St. John's Wort.

Psychoanalytic or Dynamic psychotherapy—Unlike the other forms of psychotherapy that focus on present behavior, this treatment attempts to address deeply rooted internal conflicts and residual trauma from past events that are believed to be the root cause of depressive symptoms. This peeling back of layer after layer of memory and thought typically is accomplished over years of regular visits with a therapist. The investment of time and money is questionable, however, since psychoanalysis is not a well studied treatment for major depression.

Each of the above therapies may be conducted individually or in groups. Although many people initially feel more comfortable in individual treatment, group therapies are nearly as effective for those who are able to "take the plunge."

Is there any kind of mood disorder that shouldn't be treated with psychotherapy?

An all-out ban on any one treatment is not common; however, there are some treatments that work so much better than psychotherapy for a given disorder that doctors who don't recommend them risk their reputations and/or malpractice charges. For instance, I would never suggest using psychotherapy alone for the treatment of bipolar disorder or a psychotic-depressive episode. Drug therapy is clearly called for in these situations, although it may be used in conjunction with some form of psychological counseling or therapy. The more severe an episode of major depression, the less likely it will respond well to psychotherapies; again, I would try anti-depressants for these cases first, either alone or in combination with therapy, unless a patient is vehemently opposed to the use of chemical options. If you haven't responded to psychotherapy after eight to twelve weeks, ask your doctor for a referral to someone who can help you explore drug options. That doesn't mean you have to stop the behavioral training if it appeals to you, just that it may be more successful when it's given a chemical boost.

Does psychotherapy work?

Yes! But it also depends on the patient, the particular mood disorder involved, and the quality of the service provided. There seems little question that people benefit from psychotherapy compared to those who never receive treatment. One recent study tracking patients over a period of 6 months observed an improvement in symptoms in 50 percent of patients after just eight weeks, and 75 percent of patients after six months. And, if you compare the numbers to those of people using pharmacotherapy, the drugs only win in terms of the speed of response. Used in combination, though, these two treatments produce better results than just drug therapy alone for more severe or recurrent depressions, so psychotherapy definitely has some positive effects.

Some forms are more effective for individuals than others—even cultural factors play a role in this treatment's success. For instance, for some cultures, psychotherapies designed to foster self-esteem through vigorous empowerment exercises are frightening or absurd. Women or minorities experiencing routine prejudice may benefit from therapies which focus on building positive self-images and establishing more efficient coping mechanisms for stressful social interactions. Psychotherapies like IPT typically work very well for such patients alone or in tandem with drug treatment. These special populations should look for a therapist who is culturally sensitive, either through training or personal background.

If depression is chemical, why does psychotherapy help?

Think of it this way: If you suddenly heard gunshots outside your doctor's office, you would have a chemical response—things would happen in your body, that could be recorded—your heart rate would speed up, breathing might quicken, brain waves might peak for a moment. But if your doctor had warned you, "In a minute, you'll hear gunshots because they are filming a movie down the corridor," your reactions would be far less than if you hadn't been prepared. Your body's chemical responses would not have been the same because your mind's response wouldn't have carried the same meaning. That's a very basic example of how a physiological response can be influenced by the meaning a person brings to an experience. But it may help you understand how meaning is ultimately translated into how cells chemically "talk" to each other.

In addition, physical well-being can be modified by behavioral activities—think of the positive effects of aerobic exercise, diet, and weight loss on high blood pressure or diabetes. The repetitive thought "I am worthless" has very depressing implications. Discussing areas of worth and accomplishment, engaging in diversionary activities that bolster mood, or learning to challenge negative thinking can indeed alter brain activity.

I have put my family through so much with my awful anxiety attacks. Can family therapy really help them, too, or is it just another crutch for me?

If, indeed, your family has been put through the wringer along with you, then family therapy might be a helpful component of your treatment plan. Anxiety and depression can put a significant strain on family function. Of course, this method of therapy is not for every family and is not usually a first-choice treatment for depression. But if your family life has been profoundly affected by a member's illness, if symptoms are putting a marriage at risk, or if your family is somehow contributing toward a deterioration of coping skills, it may be a good option.

How about light-based therapy? Does it work for other kinds of depression beside seasonal affective disorder?

So far, there is no evidence that phototherapy is effective in the treatment of any disorder other than the winter depression (seasonal pattern) forms of recurrent major depression and bipolar disorder. Light therapy, as it is sometimes called, usually involves exposure to a full-spectrum fluorescent light source for a period of up two hours a day. Full-spectrum lamps used for this purpose are generally 12 times brighter than those commonly found in homes (measured as Lux, a phototherapy light box generates up to 10,000 Lux at a distance of three feet, compared to a 100–200 Lux output from a lamp). Sessions can become expensive, considering the time involved, and your health-insurance provider may not subsidize the cost of the light box (i.e., $300–$600 is typical). If phototherapy is not an option financially, you could try St. John's Wort. Think of other home "remedies" that might help, like: cutting back tree branches that shade your windows from winter sun; removing heavy curtains or replacing them with ones sheer enough to let in light; making sure you go outdoors for an hour or so around noon, when light is brightest. Scheduling your vacations for midwinter and traveling to a sunny spot will help, too. Also, keep in mind that winter depressions also respond to antidepressant medications.

What is electric shock therapy? It sounds like some form of torture.

Don't worry; this therapy is far from torturous, although when people use that old term it certainly does sound scary. The more accurate name for this treatment is electroconvulsive therapy, or ECT, and it is the most effective short-term approach to the treatment of severe depression or for depressions deemed "refractory"—those particularly resistant to drug therapy. ECT has gotten a raw deal in the media, however, since most popular images of it reflect the practice dating back to a time when the therapy was far cruder and less targeted. Nowadays, ECT is essentially painless and only temporarily disorienting. Although treatment often begins in the hospital, it now frequently shifts to an outpatient basis.

Here's how the therapy works: a patient is first given a series of tests such as X-rays, heart monitoring, and blood and urine analysis to determine that it is safe to use the electrical stimulus of ECT. Electrodes are applied briefly to specific spots on the head and patients are sedated while the procedure is taking place. Once asleep, patients receive electrical impulses that alter brain waves. A seizure is induced in the brain, but the body no longer experiences the tonic-clonic jerks of a grand mal convulsion. When patients wake, they may be disoriented or confused for a short while, but quickly recover.

Between eight and twelve treatments are needed to complete a course of ECT, administered in a period far shorter than antidepressants and St. John's Wort need to begin their work. For this reason, ECT is the best option for people who require rapid treatment for their depression. It's also a drug-free alternative for pregnant women and nursing mothers with severe mood disorder, who should probably not be using St. John's Wort, either.

Is ECT scary for those who use it? Perhaps the first time, as with any new therapy, but most people treated this way report ECT is no more troubling an experience than a routine visit to the dentist. The treatment is successful for about 80 percent of those who try it. The downside is that some people do experience memory problems for months after therapy, although there is little evidence of permanent effects. ECT has *no* known irreversible effects on the brain—this has its downside, too, since relapse of depression is therefore inevitable. Unless drug therapy is used in the continuation phase following ECT, there is at least a 50 percent risk for relapse during the first year.

What could happen if I don't use any kind of treatment—not even St. John's Wort?

If you are suffering from single-episode major depression and decide to "wait out" your symptoms, chances are they will last no more than nine to twelve months. That may sound "doable" but think of it: since depression's effects are felt virtually every day of that period, you are probably looking at somewhere between 270 and 365 days of misery. But let's say you make it through the episode. If you didn't get treatment for this initial event, chances are about fifty–fifty you'll experience a relapse within the next few years. Compare that to a figure like 10 to 20 percent, which is your low-risk factor if you stay on treatment for at least six months after the acute phase.

Chronic depression, such as is seen in dysthymia, usually does not go away by itself. Even if a major depression disorder runs its typical course and tapers off after a number of months, a lot of irretrievable damage will have been done: depression's toll on your family life, love and friendship relationships, and work productivity may be already taken. Will your family be able to forget the pain you put them through as you struggled without therapeutic support? Will your boss forgive the days absent or inefficient performance? Will you ever really be able to make up for that time in terms of lost pleasure?

Then there's the even more serious scenario. Suicide is a much higher risk for those who do not seek help in coping with their condition. It is one of the leading causes of death, upping the ante in all age groups.

How can I guarantee successful treatment?

You know this already: There are no guarantees in life besides death and taxes. But you can do things to make your therapy more effective and increase its chances for success:

1. Stick to it and follow through—conscientiously complete the full course
2. Take it seriously
3. Keep records about the therapy—doses taken, how you're feeling on the treatment, what kind of progress you have seen, if any
4. Keep a dialogue going between you and your doctor—report any changes in your condition, talk over your feelings about and responses to the condition and its treatment, and encourage your doctor to share any new information on the disorder
5. Give it time to work—don't give up when you don't see results overnight, because you *won't* see them; drug therapies typically take six to eight weeks to have an effect
6. Don't judge your success against another's—remember, your chemistry, psychology, and expression of the disorder are unique

What can I do to help my wife, who has been diagnosed with depression?

There are a number of things family members and friends can do to support a loved one suffering from mood disorder. First and foremost is learning more about the disorder, so you won't make the common mistake of telling her she should cheer up and snap out of it. Some other ways you can help people with depression and other mood disturbances:

Emotional Support

Listen

Talk truth when delusions or simple negative thoughts distort reality

Offer positive feedback on their progress in treatment

Emphasize the great things about them and point out the positive in any given situation

Try not to judge or use pejorative language like "weak" or "helpless"

Act as their advocate during encounters with skeptics or in situations where their condition has to be explained

Medical Support

Encourage them to get diagnosed and treated

Help them monitor drug therapy by keeping an eye out for side effects and reminding them to take medication if a dose is missed

Assume talk about suicide is serious, try to encourage dialogue about these feelings and let doctors know what's going on

Go along with them to doctors and therapists, preparing lists of questions and making sure they're answered

Advocate compliance with therapy, gently pushing them to continue if they begin to slide in their treatment

Active Support

Invite them out, gently persisting past initial rejection of offers (Carefully gauge the amount of pressure you apply—give them a boost not a shove)

Reintroduce them to the activities, places and people they used to enjoy

Finally, be aware that depression takes a toll on those who care for people diagnosed with the condition. Give yourself some attention, too, spending time on yourself and fulfilling your needs. You don't want to become vulnerable to depression yourself.

Are there other alternative therapies for depression besides St. John's Wort?

There are a number of therapies that are generally considered "alternative" which might be helpful in the treatment of more mild forms of depression. Some of these are actually less unconventional than you might believe, and are frequently recommended by medical doctors to their patients now. A number of them are being acknowledged by health-insurance companies as cost-effective preventative measures, and so are accepted for reimbursement under established insurance plans. Few documented studies exist to support the effectiveness of many of these alternative therapies; in some cases anecdotal evidence is all there is. So, this isn't an endorsement of one or all the treatments, just a list of the ones you might encounter in your research into alternative options:

- *Bodywork*—massage therapy that targets areas of extreme muscle tension
- *Guided Imagery/Creative Visualization*—a set of relaxation exercises designed to relieve tension and promote more positive thinking
- *Aromatherapy*—the use of concentrated oils from aromatic plants to produce sensations of calm and clarity
- *Biofeedback*—a relatively widely accepted therapy, it uses sensors attached painlessly to pulse points and other input centers on your body to record physical responses to focused thought—messages along the lines of "I am slowing my heart rate"; patients learn how to control certain body functions and brain waves, promoting relaxation and smoother body function
- *Music Therapy*—just what it sounds like; using gentle music selections to induce a state of trancelike serenity
- *Deep Breathing/Meditation*—practiced control of breathing rhythms releases tension and regulates oxygen levels in the blood; these also help refocus thought away from pain

- *Yoga*—breathing and stretching exercises that induce relaxation and enhance physical well-being
- *Nutritional Therapy*—some nutritionists believe that increasing amounts of some of the B vitamins, folic acid, vitamin C and biotin will help raise mood; other benefits are promoted through the consumption of a well-balanced diet low in sugars and caffeine; therapy may also include the increased intake of foods high in tyrosine, tryptophan, and phenylalanine is sometimes recommended.
- *Herbs*—medicinal plants other than St. John's Wort you might run across in the treatment of depression include evening primrose oil, basil, oats, lady's slipper, mugwort, lavender, black cohosh, vervain, valerian, and wood betony
- *Acupuncture/Acupressure*—the application of very fine needles or gentle pressure to very specific spots on your body that correspond to organs and other centers affected by disease; when done correctly by reputable practitioners it is not painful, though at times uncomfortable

Is there anything I can do to help "treat" my depression myself, besides take St. John's Wort?

I don't recommend self-treating even mild depression without a diagnosis and some guidance from a qualified physician. But if you're looking for ways to help yourself through this period, there are many behavioral changes and minor adjustments to lifestyle that will make a positive impact on depression:

- Give yourself a break—don't push yourself to make a difficult decision or take on a heavy burden of responsibility when you're also struggling with depression.
- Set more achievable goals—if you're facing a big challenge, break it down into a series of smaller objectives.
- Put off big decisions if you can—try not to change jobs, enter a new phase in a relationship, or even get a drastically new haircut. If you must make a decision about work, marriage, or finances, talk to a trusted friend or counselor who can help you view all sides of the issue with some kind of detachment.
- Do things you enjoy—see movies that have gotten rave

reviews, pick up an old hobby that gave you pleasure, join friends when they go out even if your first response is to say "no." But don't expect too much—we're basing success here on how you would have felt at home, not based on your "old self" or everybody else.

- Exercise—low-impact aerobic exertion helps achieve higher levels of energy and strength, with an accompanying boost to self-esteem. Exercise also may elicit the release of depression-fighting biochemicals like endorphins.
- Seek out other people—you may feel like crawling into a hole but being around others will actually make you feel better.
- Try not to set yourself up for failure or judge yourself when something you do isn't successful—remind yourself it's not just you, it could have happened to anyone.
- Cry—it's one of "nature's ways" of coping and 85 percent of women report feeling better after a good weep.
- Talk—but also listen. Don't monopolize the conversation. Elevate your focus above your own misery.
- Establish regular sleeping patterns and try to keep to them—disturbed sleep rhythms make you more vulnerable.
- Keep an informal journal—it will help you track the disorder and provide an outlet for emotions in flux.
- Laugh more—read humorous books or cartoon collections. Rent comedy videos. Look for joke pages on-line. Don't just watch sad movies and listen to melancholy songs.
- Don't skip meals—eat a balanced diet at routine intervals. This is another pattern that can impact on depression.
- Use an alternative form of birth control if you're taking oral contraceptives—this will cut down on estrogen peaks and valleys.
- Clean your office or home—top to bottom. If that's too hard, pick a corner. Come back later and do another corner. Even a "ninety-eight-pound weakling" can move a boulder with a jackhammer and a wheelbarrow. If that's too hard, get help. Work side by side with someone.
- Put on music that makes you want to dance—then dance.
- Recognize your achievements—if it's hard for you to see

　your positive accomplishments and attributes, ask a friend
　to make a list for you.
* Breathe—take deep breaths. Breathing exercises will im-
　prove oxygen levels, and focusing on rhythms is a dis-
　traction.
* Plant a low-maintenance garden.
* Create a sanctuary in your home and office—a small, se-
　rene area that may hold a photo or object that has positive
　associations; music that soothes you; colors that make you
　feel happy.

Conventional therapies or St. John's Wort—how do I choose?

It's mostly a matter of severity. If your depression is moderate to severe or you are happy with your response to current
treatment, I'd think long and hard before opting for an herbal
remedy instead. If you have bipolar disorder, highly recurrent
depression, or any psychotic symptoms, definitely steer clear
of alternative therapies and see a doctor. If, however, your
depression is diagnosed as mild, the herb might be a good first
line of defense. Before you choose, read the following chapter
to find out more about the use of St. John's Wort in depression
therapy, its potential side effects, dosing levels, and studies
done on its effectiveness. Then consider, must this be an ei-
ther/or decision? Why not use the herbal remedy to support
your treatment with other therapies, or to relieve the stress of
drug withdrawal or wash-out (the period between different
drug therapies when your system is getting rid of the last rem-
nants of the drug). St. John's Wort seems to have a place in
the treatment of less extreme mood disorder, but it doesn't
have to be at the expense of other therapies that might help,
too.

No matter what treatment you choose, or even if you decide
to delay treatment, it is important to keep track of how you
are doing. Is your depression getting better or worse? If your
symptoms aren't improving, talk with your doctor about
changing your treatment. If you aren't treating the depression,
view this lack of change as evidence that you can't delay seeking help any longer. Generally, if your depression isn't lifting,
professional treatment or a change in therapy is needed.

One way of keeping track of how you're doing is to complete the scales in Chapter 2 (pages 40–41). During treatment, you and your doctor may find it helpful to use an even simpler scale such as the following Global Rating of Improvement.

GLOBAL RATING OF IMPROVEMENT

+3   I am completely well. This is as good as it gets.

+2   I am definitely better, although not quite back to my old self.

+1   I am a little better, but this is not an acceptable amount of improvement.

 0   I am not one bit better.

−1   I am even worse than before I started treatment.

This self-help chart can be completed once a week to keep track of progress during treatment. It is adapted from the Clinician Global Impression (CGI) scale, which is widely used in depression research. A score of +2 or +3 should be obtained by the fourth or sixth week of therapy. If not, the treatment should be modified.

HOW BAD IS MY DEPRESSION?

100 I have no problem whatsoever!
│
90 My mood and functioning are really good—I
only have occasional "everyday"
│ problems.

80 I'm good, although I have an occasional
symptom *or* a little trouble at work or at
│ home.

70 I am definitely not very depressed but I do
have a few symptoms *or* some problems at
│ work or home.

60 I definitely have symptoms more days than
not *or* I have a moderate amount of
│ difficulty with my functioning.

50 I have significant symptoms *or* significant
difficulties with functioning. I definitely
│ need help!

40 and I am completely nonfunctional and
lower overwhelmed. I should seek professional
help immediately.

This scale can be administered once a week to assess overall progress. If one of the descriptions exactly matches your own self-assessment, then use the accompanying score. If not, place your score between the two descriptions that come closest to your own assessment (e.g., a score of 85, 63, or 78). It is based on a clinical research tool called the Global Assessment Scale (GAS). Most people coming for treatment of depression score between 41 and 60. Generally, an effective treatment should help you improve your rating to 70 or above. If your problems are longstanding or complicated, it may be unreasonable to expect to score 90 or 100 right away. However, it is a whole lot easier to go from 75 to 90 than to go from 50 to 90!

FOUR

❧

Is St. John's Wort Safe and Effective?

Tom sat across from his doctor, arms folded in one of his characteristic gestures, demanding to know the facts. Tom had never been one to accept anything on trust—questioning every step of the treatment process so far—and he was not about to start with some herbal remedy. So, when a friend suggested that Tom augment his depression therapy of an SSRI with St. John's Wort, he immediately made an appointment with his doctor. "I've read the 20/20 transcript," Tom reported—he spends hours searching the Internet and had found a copy on line. "I want to know—is it all true? Does this thing really work? Is it safe?" His doctor told him that there were no easy answers to his questions at the moment, and let him know about the new testing being done on the herb here in the U.S. It was not what Tom wanted to hear. "What about all these other tests I keep hearing about? Let me see what they say." Tom's therapy always worked best when he was a full partner in any decisions, so his doctor hauled out files filled with summaries of the twenty-three studies most widely mentioned in discussions of St. John's Wort. Tom struggled through the first three abstracts before throwing the pile down. "So what do they say? Can this help me?" His doctor was pretty sure, in fact, that the answer was yes. At the least it was worth a try. Tom's depression was relatively mild, and he has responded well to very low doses of

133

*medicine. But Tom needed to be involved in the decision,
as his doctor realized. They spent the rest of the session
talking about the herb. Tom's doctor summarized the
research. They discussed the information Tom had found
on-line about the herb. His doctor gave Tom some written materials to take home on herbal remedies and St.
John's Wort. Tom called four days later. "Let's do it."
He started on St. John's Wort three weeks ago; for now
it is "wait and see."*

The patients who talk to me about St. John's Wort all ask
the same two questions, even if they are presented in a dozen
different guises: Is the herb safe? Is it effective? The worse
the depression, the less emphasis they tend to place on the
former question. Risk is weighed differently when pain becomes intolerable.

The answers to these questions still aren't one hundred percent clear, and what we do know must be judged by each
patient/doctor team, just as Tom and I looked at the data from
many angles. Certainly, there is a tremendous volume of evidence—both clinical and anecdotal—to suggest the herb is
effective in the treatment of milder forms of depression.

Three million prescriptions a year are written for St. John's
Wort pills in Germany. The herb was approved as an antidepressant medicine in that country back in 1984 by the German
version of our Food and Drug Administration (Commission
E). It is also an approved therapy there for some sleep and
anxiety disorders. St. John's Wort does not enjoy the same
status here in the U.S., however, where it is only allowed to
bear the label "nutritional supplement." The reason is that
our own FDA, as well as scientists and researchers in the medical community, do not believe that the results of the tests
conducted in Germany were definitive. What are their concerns?

- Existing studies were not long enough to monitor reliably
  late-emerging side effects or determine for what period
  the extract was effective.
- The studies often did not use standard methods for measuring the type and degree of depression, and alleviation
  of symptoms, so no universally acceptable standard can

be applied and compared.

- No study has yet definitively answered questions about effective doses—how little is too little and how much too much, connections between severity of side effects and doses, and which populations or disorders should be targeted with a given amount.
- In cases where St. John's Wort's effects were compared to synthetic antidepressants, the drugs used were older-variety tricyclics (among the more side-effect-prone antidepressant medications), in doses lower than those commonly prescribed here in the U.S., making the comparisons questionable.
- The herb's actions have not been specifically tested against severe depression, bipolar and anxiety disorders, or dysthymia.

Finally, many of the European studies were not performed as double-blind trials, tests in which neither patients nor the doctors know who is working with any given substance—herb, drug, or placebo—until after the study is complete. These control methods ensure results are not unduly influenced by placebo responses. Double-blind trials are the standard the U.S.

That sounds like a lot of uncertainty. But there's room for excitement and hope, too, because the results of these studies, flawed though they may be, are very encouraging for treatment of mild to moderate depression. In one journal, where 23 of the most authoritative studies were collected and analyzed, 64% of people who took St. John's Wort pills felt better. Very few experienced side effects of any kind, and most who did felt the discomfort to be mild.

Moreover, not one single death has been attributed to the herb in the 2,400-odd years that its remedies have been in use for the treatment of mental illness, cuts, burns, bruises, and an assortment of other ills. That's an impressive statistic by anyone's standards. Aspirin accounts for approximately 800 accidental deaths each year from unexpected side effects and overdoses. So far, no one is known to have died from an overdose of St. John's Wort.

What does that mean for you? Well, if you are suffering from mild to moderate depression, seasonal affective disorder, irritable bowel syndrome that seems tied to your stress response, sleep disturbances, or mild forms of anxiety disorder, St. John's Wort might be used to help you. It's not a call you should make on your own, however. Talk with your doctor. Clarify your diagnosis. Examine your treatment plan. If you're not happy with the progress shown in current therapy of your mood disorder, discuss the option of St. John's Wort with your physician. Examine all the facts you can get your hands on: results from existing studies, plans for future trials, what is missing from the data that currently prevents St. John's Wort from becoming an officially recognized treatment in the U.S. Ask your doctor to look for the latest information in medical journals. Then take what you learn about the herb and add it to what is known about you—the person considering it for therapy—reactions to other medications, openness to alternative therapies; compliance with prior therapy routines, and, most importantly, the unique expression of the individual mood disorder.

You and your doctor need to collect and discuss the information about yourself, but what you'll find in this chapter are the latest facts about the herb, as documented in clinical studies and supported by anecdotal information. This information will provide a basis upon which you and your doctor can make an informed decision: Is St. John's Wort safe *for you*? Could it be effective *for you*?

Is St. John's Wort a cure?

St. John's Wort is not a cure. At present, there is no "cure" for depression, but treatments that alleviate its symptoms and suppress what appear to be its associated effects on the brain. St. John's Wort is a treatment for depression. How successful a treatment it will prove to be for any individual depends on a number of complex factors.

I've heard from dozens of people that this herb works. But I know I shouldn't believe everything I hear. Is it stupid to rely on the recommendations of people who aren't doctors?

Are these "dozens of people" individuals you trust for a medical opinion? Are they speaking from experience or just passing along what they have "heard" on the grapevine? The reliability of anecdotal evidence is only as good as its source, so apply a healthy helping of skepticism to any accounts of medical miracles you heard second- and thirdhand. By all means listen to what they have to say, then try to uncover the cold, hard facts through research and discussions with your doctor. What's the very latest clinical information out there?

It is true that millions of people have been using the herb in Germany, and many millions more have used it in some way, shape or form through the twenty-four-odd centuries of its recorded use. But this anecdotal evidence, while weighty, is just one of the factors you should consider. Others include: Are their life and health situations close to your own? Were all these people using the same doses? Did the dose have an effect on their success in treating depression? Did any other elements have an impact? Exactly what levels of depression and anxiety were helped by the herbal remedy? These questions cannot be answered in any accurate, cohesive way through anecdotal information alone. They need to be addressed in studies using carefully documented criteria and controls. Base your decisions about therapies on a range of sources—both trustworthy anecdotes and clinical conclusions.

Is there any scientific proof that St. John's Wort works?

There have been literally dozens of studies examining the effectiveness of St. John's Wort as a treatment for depressive illness, some more reliable than others and most conducted abroad. Among other things, these studies have compared the herb's effects against placebos and low doses of prescription-drug treatments. Overall, St. John's Wort was shown to be significantly better at resolving mild depression than the placebos and had about the same effectiveness as the drugs tested. Depending on the study, success rates hover at between 40 and 80%. The higher numbers come from uncontrolled trials, so a placebo response might account for the marked increase.

I hear all about these "European" studies, but isn't there any research being done on St. John's Wort here in the U.S.?

In the past, no; St. John's Wort was not a popular subject for clinical studies in the U.S. The recent explosion of interest in St. John's Wort in this country no doubt spurred the decision by some major players to initiate new studies into the effectiveness of St. John's Wort as a treatment for depression. Together, the National Institutes of Health's Office of Alternative Medicine (OAM), The National Institute for Mental Health (NIMH), and the Office of Dietary Supplements (ODS) were funding research on the subject as this book was being written (see more about this study later in the chapter).

What were the results of all those studies I've been hearing about?

The study you are mostly likely to encounter in your research into St. John's Wort—and the one typically quoted by media reports on the herb—was actually a review of data from a collection of many separate clinical trials, a "meta-analysis," which addressed concerns about drawing conclusion from small-scale studies by combining results from many on the same subject, allowing for broader summations to be drawn. In this meta-analysis, twenty-three such studies (twenty of them double-blind) were collected, reviewed, and published in the August 3, 1996, issue of the *British Medical Journal*. In that article, entitled "St. John's Wort for depression—An overview and meta-analysis of randomized clinical trials," results were examined encompassing 1,757 outpatients, most described as having mild to moderate levels of depression disorder. The conclusion drawn by that overview pretty much sums up both the hopeful nature of many such study results of St. John's Wort to date and the reason why these studies are still not considered definitive by our own medical establishment and the FDA:

> There is evidence that extracts of Hypericum perforatum are more effective than placebo for the treatment of mild to moderately severe depressive disorders. Further studies comparing extracts with standard antidepressants in well defined groups of patients and comparing different extracts and doses are needed.

The overview noted that 64% of the subjects tallied in the studies felt markedly better compared to 59% receiving synthetic antidepressants. Only 4% of those receiving St. John's

Wort therapy dropped out because of side effects, while 8% taking the antidepressant drugs discontinued their treatment.

Just how popular is St. John's Wort in Germany?

Does 66 million doses a year sound popular? That's how much St. John's Wort was consumed by German patients in 1994. How about 200,000 prescriptions *per month*? If those numbers don't convey the herb's popularity, compare its sales to that of Prozac, which averages just 30,000 prescriptions per month. In Germany, St. John's Wort is the most commonly used antidepressant therapy.

Here in the U.S. 20 million doses of Prozac are prescribed each year. When you consider that many of these people might shift over to an herbal remedy, you can see why pharmaceutical companies might not be rushing to supply money for a clinical study—unless they somehow manage to figure out a process for standardizing whatever St. John's Wort active ingredients turn out to be, in an extract of consistent quality (hypericin is just a guess so far, and standardizing the herb to its contents appears to be having some positive effect). Pharmaceutical companies do have a positive model, however. Despite the fact that it can be purchased over the counter in Germany, 80% of all sales of St. John's Wort in that country come from prescriptions, no doubt because such purchases are reimbursed under their current health-care system.

If there have been all these tests already on St. John's Wort and so many people are using it in Germany, why are doctors here still worried that it isn't safe?

For many years, doctors were concerned because not enough patients were studied in any given study to draw definitive conclusions, even in those studies abroad. While more recent trials have tracked larger populations of patients (one involved over 1,700 depression sufferers), many researchers in the U.S. remain skeptical about the reliability of such studies performed abroad because the criteria used typically don't meet the rigorous standards required by our own medical society or the FDA. Basic data-collecting standards here require researchers make no definite conclusions until the results of clinical trials are re-

peated several times, with the same effects, using large populations—to estimate better the substance's actions in a wide array
of people and on very well-defined conditions. Moreover, doctors and federal regulators want to see results drawn from
longer-term trials. Most studies stopped tracking patients after
four or six weeks of use. Though some people in Europe have
been using the herb for years, our own regulatory agencies have
learned a "better safe than sorry" approach after the failures of
thalidomide and other apparent "miracle" drugs proved dangerous in the long term. Also, as more becomes known about
the herb more people are more likely to make connections between actions, adverse effects, and their own (often not
physician-monitored) use of the herb. A recent case reported by
a doctor in the popular press might be the first noted incident of
serious illness associated with St. John's Wort—a case of stroke
in an elderly patient being treated for a bladder condition—or it
may prove to have nothing to do with the herb after all (one current theory holds that the patient's doses of St. John's Wort
were adulterated in some way that proved dangerous to an
already-weakened older patient).

How does St. John's Wort fight depression?

Various of the herb's constituents are thought to have an
effect: Hypericin and pseudohypericin may be the ones you
hear about most often, but researchers are now coming to believe that other constituents—like hyperforin, polycyclic phe-
nols (with its subclass of flavonoids such as rutin, quercitin,
and quercetin), kaempferol, and luteolin—may also be at work
on depression. Some theorists believe it is not one of these
agents working alone, but some combination of two or more
of them.

But the latest theory gaining favor is that one flavonoid,
amentoflavone, may be the agent most responsible for St.
John's Wort's antidepressant effects. It appears to be effective
in this action by binding receptors, which alters the signals
between cells triggered by neurotransmitters.

No one knows precisely what the herb's actions are in the
treatment of depression. Instead, there are mostly questions
with only partial answers, some of which are discussed more
fully elsewhere in this chapter:

- Does St. John's Wort act as a monoamine oxidase inhibitor? Almost certainly, but probably not to the extent previously thought—and, surprisingly, not by way of hypericin but more likely through the actions of flavonoids.
- What about the herb's serotonin-reuptake inhibition? There is probably some of that happening as well, but again not at a level potent enough to work on its own.
- Is St. John's Wort a catechol-O-methyltransferase (COMT) inhibitor, preventing this enzyme from breaking down pleasure-producing amines? More and more researchers suspect this action is involved, but again COMT inhibitors are not as widely researched as antidepressants.
- Does it change sleep patterns, reversing the damage done to circadian rhythms by depression? It looks like St. John's Wort might, indeed, improve the quality of sleep.
- Is St. John's Wort shifting hormonal pathways by stopping the release of various interleukins? The herbal remedy just may be involved in slowing this protein's actions, preventing an overenthusiastic immune response.
- Is there an estrogen connection, or some relationship to other hormones? It seems likely, from a few tests conducted on rodents and the presence of one agent, betasitosterol.
- Does St. John's Wort alter dopamine levels in the brain? It now looks like St. John's Wort may increase dopamine action by working on the neurotransmitter gamma-aminobutyric acid.

Most researchers believe that St. John's Wort works on depression because some combination of its agents target all these diverse effects—just as some doctors now suspect a wide variety of chemical causes are behind depression's manifold effects.

I've heard St. John's Wort changes rhythms in your brain that control sleep. Will it help with my insomnia?

There is some indication that St. John's Wort has an impact on circadian rhythms, the body's pattern of regular cycles such as eating, body temperature, and, of course, sleep. The most definitive information of St. John's Wort's relationship to sleep cycles comes from a German study of brain-wave activity in older subjects. It was shown that St. John's Wort had little effect on REM cycles, the period of rapid eye movement sleep during which dreaming takes place. By contrast, SSRIs, tricyclics, and MAOIs have been shown to affect this phase of sleep. St. John's Wort likewise did not alleviate insomnia— it did not modify the subjects' inability to fall asleep or stay asleep if that was the problem. Instead, the herbal remedy appeared to deepen the *level* of sleep during periods when a person was able to rest. In another test conducted in Germany, using an extract commercially available in that country named Hyperforat, melatonin levels were shown to increase during sleep. Melatonin is a hormone implicated in controlling sleep cycles that is itself produced in greater quantities during the evening hours prior to slumber. One word of warning, however: Insomnia was a side effect of the herb mentioned in some of the European clinical trials. So it appears the herb can have either a beneficial or negative effect on insomnia.

Is St. John's Wort an MAOI? An SSRI? A COMT-inhibitor?

Because we don't know exactly how St. John's Wort works on depression, researchers are, at the moment, largely relying on comparisons to synthetic antidepressants classified with these actions to determine whether the herb is one of these or some combination.

An MAOI is a substance that stops (inhibits) a particular type of enzyme (monoamine oxidase, or MAO) from performing its functions. Some of these functions of MAO are to break down (metabolize) dopamine, epinephrine, norepinephrine, and serotonin after they have completed their jobs as neurotransmitters, processing their messages of pain or pleasure, among other things. For a long time St. John's Wort was thought to be an MAOI and hypericin the agent most likely responsible for these actions. But more recent studies, notably one published in the October 1997 issue of the *Journal of Geriatric Psychiatry and Neurology*, concluded this is not the case by isolating hypericin and observing its solo effects. Another study used higher levels of hypericin and other constituents in rats; no corresponding decline in the levels of MAO was observed. It concluded that *Hypericum*'s antidepressant effects could not be explained in terms of MAO inhibition. That is not to say monoamine oxidase or serotonin does not play a role, only that MAOI inhibitory activity alone can't explain the herbal remedy's impact on depression. One source on the herb, an FAQ (frequently-asked questions) produced by registered nurse Camilla Cracchiolo, reminds us that these tests were made using liquid extracts of St. John's Wort, and calls into question whether whole-herb products are as free of MAOI actions. It is possible (although unlikely) that the agent with MAOI effects is not soluble in the liquids, like alcohol, that are used for extracts. See the section on side effects on page 147 for more information about St. John's Wort and the debate over its relationship to this enzyme's functions.

SSRIs, or serotonin-reuptake inhibitors, also impede the cells' efforts to "cleanup," but act on the neurotransmitter site that helps take up (or reuptake), in this case specifically, serotonin back into the cell. But St. John's Wort is not an SSRI, either; it is not selective in its effects and does not potently block serotonin reuptake.

Another study looked at COMT-inhibiting actions. COMT is an acronym for catechol-O-methyltransferase, a natural enzyme that alters the body's production of the neurotransmitters dopamine, epinephrine, and norepinephrine. These are all players in the feelings of energy, pleasure and pain. Flavonols and xanthones in St. John's Wort may have COMT-inhibiting effects, but that has not been definitively established.

I've heard that the reason hypericin works is because it can cross the "blood-brain barrier." What is that?

Capillaries are tiny blood vessels that carry oxygen-rich blood from the arteries to the tissues then return the nutrient-depleted blood back to the veins. Many exchanges of chemical substances occur during this exchange because capillary walls are thin enough to allow certain substances to pass through them—all except capillaries in the brain. There, a sort of barrier shield exists, a hurdle to substances that might harm the brain or impede its functions. This barrier is determined by just how "fat soluble" a substance is; the more soluble, the easier to get access to brain cells.

But that protection has its downside—some substances that

could help the brain fight disease or dysfunction, such as medications, have a hard time getting through, too. Some agents
in St. John's Wort may be able to cross this microscopic barrier. It has been hinted at in studies but never significantly
explored.

Is it true you risk serious burns if you go out in the sun while taking St. John's Wort?

Even the most enthusiastically pro-*Hypericum* articles and
postings I've encountered mention photosensitive reaction as
a potential, albeit rare, side effect of treatment with St. John's
Wort. Phototoxicity is, in reality, *so* rare a symptom only one
case has been officially documented in a person taking any
form of the natural herb remedy in normal therapeutic dosages—that of an elderly woman who had been using the herbal
remedy in her depression therapy for over 3 years, who developed itching, rashlike lesions. This reaction reversed itself
when St. John's Wort treatment was stopped. I have noted an
occasional anecdotal report, generally secondhand, of someone
getting a bad sunburn from brief sun exposure while taking
St. John's Wort, but I would not base a general caution against
this side effect on the basis of such thin documentation. In any
event, whatever modest risk that might be faced can be min-
imized by limiting sun exposure and using a good sunblock.

Originally, concern about this side effect arose from reports
of illness and even fatality among livestock grazing on the
herb. Those animals were suffering from an effect termed photosensitization, a reaction that caused them to become abnormally sensitive to sun exposure. Photosensitization occurs
when hypericin is improperly absorbed through the intestines
and makes its way to the skin. Sunlight alters the chemical
and the body reacts with an allergic response.

Such an effect was noted as early as 1787 and became so inextricably associated with the herb, the chemical alteration is
occasionally called "hypericism," and in Russia the herb's
common name can be roughly translated as "beast-killer." It is
also one of the reasons why ranchers both in the U.S. and Australia consider the herb a plant pest. Photosensitization in livestock presents itself as painful burns and sores on their skin.
Prolonged exposure and infection led to some fatalities among
those animals. Remember, though, livestock consume vast

quantities of the herb as they graze, in amounts far higher than any normal "human" doses of the herb. Too, the effects of photosensitization were not observed in lab tests conducted on other animal species, except predator insects. It appears that the massive amounts consumed by livestock and insects, coupled with the ruminant characteristic of cattle, who pass food through their stomachs in a way different than other species, may have affected their photosensitization response to St. John's Wort.

Despite the fact that humans seem protected from this effect, fear spurred by the cattle fatalities led to placement of St. John's Wort on the FDA's list of "unsafe" herbs in 1977, making it illegal to sell the herbal extract. It wasn't until a new dietary law was enacted in 1984, which required the FDA to prove danger definitively before placing a ban, that the herb was returned to store shelves in the U.S. At about that time, St. John's Wort was approved for therapeutic use in Germany. In the years that followed more data about photosensitization (or rather a pronounced *lack* of data) was compiled. Among the many millions of people who have since used the drug in Europe, Asia, and Canada, no sun-toxic effects have been reported by physicians. Even an active rumor mill has produced only a tiny handful of anecdotal reports of mild burns. In the U.S., a small number of unofficial accounts describe a reaction akin to a bad sunburn or skin rashes in very light-skinned people—a temporary response that ceased when treatment with the herbal remedy was stopped. Most often, those reporting such effects were using St. John's Wort as a therapy for their infection with HIV. In an attempt to mimic the high levels of concentrated synthetic hypericin used in clinical trials on AIDS, these individuals were using doses many times in excess of those utilized in depression therapy. One study estimates normal therapeutic doses for depression are thirty to fifty times below the levels which promote phototoxicity.

Fears about this extraordinarily rare side effect persist, however, despite the volume of evidence that risk is negligible. These fears were given a boost a few years ago when one AIDS-related clinical trial had to be stopped when a few volunteers demonstrated severe photosensitive reactions—rashes, and an inability to tolerate sunlight for more than fifteen minutes without the appearance of swelling, redness, and facial pain. What is not often repeated in warnings that mention this failed trial is the fact that the substance being used was not a normal dose of plant-based extract, but a synthetic extract—the first such man-made "replica" of concentrated hypericin to be tested on humans. The hypericin was administered in high doses and taken intravenously. Other patients in the study who took the same extract in an oral dose were not similarly affected. Generally, medications given intravenously reach much higher concentration than those taken orally.

Finally, results of another test relating to photosensitization haven't received the same dissemination as rumors surrounding the aborted trial of synthetic hypericin. This other clinical trial was focused on the side effect; researchers actually attempted to provoke a phototoxic response. Subjects were given essentially double the dose normally administered in depression therapy—600 mg three times daily—for 15 days. No photosensitization took place in any of the volunteers, despite higher-than-normal hypericin levels in the blood.

In the face of this evidence, this is clearly not a side effect to fear. Yet doctors and herbalists who have not read all the literature still opt to remain on the safe side, prompting light-skinned patients to wear long-sleeved clothing, hats, and sunscreen and limit direct exposure to the sun while on a therapy that uses the herb. Perhaps that's not so bad, as these precautions are recommended pretty routinely these days, in light of what we know about the potential for skin cancers as a result of prolonged sun exposure. My opinion, though, is that the theoretical risk of photosensitization is so slight it should not prevent persons otherwise eligible from using St. John's Wort in their depression treatment.

I've heard that St. John's Wort is photodynamic. Do I need to sit in the sun for it to work on my depression?

This is the flip side of the photosensitization coin, but is an area that needs to be further explored. In the lab, hypericin extracts have been radiated with light prior to their administration in antiviral and cancer-fighting (antineoplastic) studies. The herb's effects were clearly enhanced in these actions by first being exposed to light in the form of radiation. The herb's relationship to light comes as no surprise to some. St. John's Wort folklore is suffused with images of the sun.

Herbalists typically warn people to keep dried herbs away

from the sun but also note that liquid extractions need daily doses of light as they are processed, to preserve the strength of the herb's volatile oils and other active agents. How this light exposure works in depression therapy is less clearly understood. Still, some patients find regular exposure to light seems to help the herb's effects. This will most probably prove to be a factor when the herb's actions on cases of seasonal affective disorder are examined more closely.

I've heard St. John's Wort has *no* side effects. Can that possibly be right?

No medication, however benign, has absolutely no potential side effects. Many people actually experience side effects from substances most people would consider perfectly harmless—vitamins, minerals and supplements—but simply don't associate their therapies with the mild symptoms they encounter. This typically occurs unless side effects persist or increase in intensity; most people tend to shrug milder symptoms off, often blaming them on other sources besides the remedy.

The same might be true of St. John's Wort, since typical side effects (also called adverse drug reactions or ADRs) are mild and fairly general: dry mouth, irritability, a feeling of fatigue, skin rashes, itching, stomach upset and abdominal pain, diarrhea, dizziness, loss of appetite, and nausea. I have also run across a number of anecdotal accounts of light-headedness, sleeplessness, anxiety, and nervousness. Weight gain was noted in a few people taking St. John's Wort in a mixture that includes kavakava. All documented side effects of St. John's Wort have been reversible when treatment with the herbal remedy was ended. In addition, many of the side effects mentioned in relation to St. John's Wort therapy are side effects experienced to the same or greater extents by people using antidepressant drugs—although St. John's Wort appears to be free of any negative impact on sexual function, heart rate, or the nervous system, symptoms that provoke the most dropouts from treatment in people using prescription antidepressants.

Some herbalists believe that a few of St. John's Wort's symptoms, such as stomach upset and diarrhea, are appropriate responses to herbal remedies in the first few weeks of use, claiming that this is the result of the body cleansing itself of toxins. That has not been documented, and if the symptoms are uncomfortable, you should discuss them with your doctor. And, if the side effects are disabling or worsen rather than lessen over time, I would discontinue use of the herb immediately. Where a negative response to St. John's Wort therapy is most extreme or skin rashes appear, an allergic response seems indicated.

The good news, and the basis for the overly enthusiastic claims of "no side effects" you've heard, is that the incidence of serious side effects from use of St. John's Wort appears to be very rare indeed if the herbal remedy is taken in normal doses. The number of documented occurrences of side effects both mild and severe compares favorably to that of synthetic antidepressants. In the twenty-three clinical trials collected in the often-cited *BMJ* meta-analysis of St. John's Wort studies, these were the overall results:

1,757 subjects	Subjects who experienced side effects	Subjects who dropped out because of side effects
Total number of all patients using St. John's Wort	50 or 19.8%	2 or 0.8%
Total number of all patients using synthetic antidepressants	84 or 52.8%	7 or 3.0%

Numbers were even lower in another study published in another *Journal* analysis of 6 studies:

1,757 subjects	Subjects who experienced side effects
Total number of all patients using St. John's Wort	10.8%
Total number of all patients using synthetic antidepressants	35.9%

In a study of 1,008 patients comparing St. John's Wort's effects to those of a placebo, results were interesting, too, suggesting once again that the herb's effects are not simply generated by patients' expectations of results.

1,008 subjects	Subjects who experienced side effects	Subjects who dropped out because of side effects
Total number of all patients using St. John's Wort	**4.1%**	**0.4%**
Total number of all patients on placebo	**4.8%**	**1.8%**

A large-scale study that documented effects in 3,250 patients documented that only seventy-nine of the test subjects reported unpleasant side effects and of those, only forty-eight were made uncomfortable enough to discontinue treatment of the herbal remedy. That means that only 2.4% experienced side effects at all and just 1.4% of subjects had effects they could not tolerate—a significantly small number for such a test. The study was uncontrolled—that is, no second group was examined on placebo or another therapy to compare to the herb's actions, but uncontrolled studies are still considered reliable indicators of side-effect presentation and risk. Here's how the individual symptoms broke down:

MOST COMMON SIDE EFFECTS REPORTED IN CLINICAL STUDIES	PERCENTAGE OF SUBJECTS REPORTING EFFECT
gastrointestinal irritations	0.55% of all volunteers (Remember, this figure is *point* 55 or just slightly more than ½ of 1%.)
allergic reactions	0.52%
tiredness	0.40%
restlessness	0.27%

The numbers should tell you how few people experience intolerable side effects while using St. John's Wort—but also reinforce how relatively few demonstrate debilitating effects from more conventional therapies during this early phase of treatment as well—a fact to keep in mind if your herbal therapy is unsuccessful.

How come St. John's Wort acts like a drug but doesn't have a drug's side effects?

It is possible that St. John's Wort's wide range of active chemical constituents are responsible for its relatively trouble-free effects. Each of these agents is distinct, with focused actions that, combined, target a variety of body functions. But each may be relatively moderate, having a potent impact on depression only because its forces are linked with a host of other effects. No single neurotransmitter receives a strong effect, so a kind of balance is achieved. This type of unifying approach is not matched in the narrower focus of prescription drugs, that can provoke a correspondingly sharp response.

You mean *no one* has gotten seriously ill because they used St. John's Wort?

No clinically documented cases exist. Very recently, however, I read a newly updated FAQ on the herb which mentioned three cases that may initiate more examination of St. John's Wort's side effects and drug interactions. The cases involved:

- An elderly woman being treated for bladder spasms with a prescription drug described as having the effect of "stimulating the sympathetic nervous system." Shortly after beginning treatment with St. John's Wort for depression, the woman experienced a sharp rise in blood pressure resulting in a hypertensive crisis and subsequent stroke. Such a reaction—most commonly seen when mixing MAOIs with tyramine-rich substances or drugs—might have proven fatal. As it is, the woman suffered right-side paralysis. The jury is still out on whether St. John's Wort was responsible, at what dose it was taken, or if, as seems likely, the herb was taken in its whole-herb form (which does not have the same low-MAOI effect as the extracts tested in trials) or adulterated in some way (mixing herbs with other, unidentified and unacknowledged substances is a not-uncommon practice of a few unscrupulous manufacturers whose poor practices unfairly and unfortunately give the whole herbal industry a bad name.) The case was reported in a newspaper and noted in more recent articles on St. John's Wort, but it has not been scientifically documented or data about the case officially submitted for review by experts on the herb.

• A young woman using the herb presented an unusual combination of symptoms that finally resulted in hospitalization: dizziness, fever, a feeling of faintness when standing or walking, confusion, unsteadiness, periodic hot flashes, night sweats, diarrhea, an accelerated heart rate, chest and throat spasms, shortness of breath, and high blood pressure that did not respond to treatment with beta-blocker medication. These are considered classic symptoms of serotonin syndrome, a condition in which all serotonin activity is increased excessively, producing too strong a response for your body to handle. It is rare and can be fatal if not addressed. As no other serotonin-provoking medication was being taken by the patient, doctors concluded the reaction was somehow linked to the St. John's Wort therapy she was using for depression. Again, this is not a documented case; it is a secondhand report noted in a newsletter of sorts, which itself openly admits more needs to be known about the case before drawing any correlation between St. John's Wort and serotonin syndrome. Again, it may turn out that this expression of the syndrome is not related or not the direct consequence of her use of St. John's Wort or that the dose was adulterated in some way. Certainly, millions of patients in Germany have used the herb with no such effects.

• Finally, a patient with epilepsy who had not suffered a seizure in some time was documented by his physician as experiencing a rapid succession of twenty-five seizures just days after beginning therapy with St. John's Wort. Seizures disappeared when the treatment with St. John's Wort was immediately stopped. Was the herb even involved or was the timing coincidental? Did the antiseizure medication interact adversely with the herb?

In the light of these three cases, and their lack of documentation and scrutiny thus far, it is difficult to draw any definitive conclusions about safety. Again, it becomes a balance between benefit and risk. If you are susceptible to either stroke or seizure, and are on a serotonin-enhancing medication, then you may determine that the risks, however slight (after all we are talking about three cases out of a history of millions of St. John's Wort users), outweigh the potential for success with treatment of the herb. If you have a family history of or are currently battling any serious condition, I would use caution in adding St. John's Wort to your combination of medications on general principles—more is often not merrier when it comes to medications.

Is it possible to have an allergic reaction to an herb?

Yes it is; it is possible to have an allergic reaction to *any* substance. No studies have been conducted examining allergic reactions to this particular herbal remedy—who may be more susceptible to them or what other allergies could be linked—but I have run across a few descriptions of documented side effects and anecdotal accounts that sound like allergic reaction. These were marked by more-severe-than-normal side effects experienced very soon after beginning treatment of the drug. The side effects most often demonstrated in cases like these were stomach pain, diarrhea, headache, dizziness, skin rashes, and pruritis—a persistent sensation of itching. If you have proven allergic to St. John's Wort in the past, do not attempt a second treatment with the herb. Allergic reactions do not typically go away and often become worse with each new exposure.

Aren't all natural remedies safe?

The commonly held belief that natural equals safe is a false impression that makes those in the medical field very nervous. Plants can kill—people are routinely poisoned by eating the wrong mushrooms; comfrey is an herb that may cause liver damage over time, when taken internally. Think of all the mysteries that owe their central murders to poisoning by foxglove, aka digitalis. And recall that alcohol, opium, cocaine, and to-bacco are "natural." Moreover, any substance taken in ex-cess—natural or not—has the potential to be dangerous or produce uncomfortable side effects. Too-high doses of niacin can result in severe gastrointestinal problems and end in liver damage. Continuous high intake of vitamin D may damage your kidney and promote bone deformity. The most common cause of all child poisoning deaths in the U.S. is the result of children consuming their parent's iron tablets—just 6 high-potency pills can produce serious injury. In 1989, over 1,500 cases of a connective tissue disorder called eosinophilia-myalgia syndrome (EMS) were traced to the use of supple-ments containing L-tryptophan. This illness led to thirty-eight known deaths. *Ephedra,* an herb sometimes called Ma Huang and found in many herbal dieting aids, has been linked to over 800 cases of severe side effects reported to the FDA, and also some deaths. Such "Herbal Phen-Fens," as they have become known, are universally derided by doctors and patients alike, who feel they are unsafe and should not be commercially available.

These words of caution are included because many people exploring the use of St. John's Wort may be inclined to use other supplements as well. It is a warning, too, against using the herb in any mixtures, or compounds, that include other ingredients. Even if St. John's Wort is gentle, there is no such guarantee about the other elements in the mix.

Many people in the medical, food, and herbal communities support the laws and guidelines currently being considered that address labeling of dietary supplements and other "natural" products. New rules are being enacted that would allow man-ufacturers to spell out more clearly the effects of their prod-ucts—both beneficial and negative. This would include passing on cautionary information a consumer should know about any given substance, like the risk for harmful side ef-fects, interactions, and toxic results from excessive or long-term use.

I know many Germans have been using St. John's Wort for years. Have there been any negative long-term effects?

In only one study conducted to date have patients been mon-itored for more than eight weeks and their longer-term reactions documented. So, as far as scientific evidence on the herbal remedy's effects over time is concerned—there really is no definitive answer. Plenty of anecdotal information exists on the subject, however, based on cases of German patients who have been using that country's approved therapies for the treatment of their depression for years, but these reports vary. One I ran across mentioned a patient who claimed to have used it regularly for a decade. I cannot yet recommend such prolonged use, but it is reassuring to note, from a safety standpoint, no serious illness has been recorded in Europe resulting from long-term use of St. John's Wort for depression therapy. Not one death has been connected to the herb's use so far, either. I have heard from several patients that they felt the herb's effects declined after about a year on the therapy, but we are talking about such limited numbers that no real conclusions can be drawn from them. It is clear further studies need to be made of large populations of patients who have been using the herb for long periods, with regular follow-ups to note any increase in side effects and decrease in effectiveness.

I hear you can buy it like candy over in Germany. How come?

Technically, you can buy St. John's Wort "like candy" here in the U.S., too, since you can find commercial preparations of the herb in many supermarkets and drugstores only an aisle or two away from a bagful of M&Ms. Hopefully, though, people are giving more consideration to the purchase of St. John's Wort—or any other herbal remedy—than they give to their choice of a chocolate or gum. The stories you've heard about its accessibility probably reflect a reaction to the fact that St. John's Wort is used by millions of people in Europe for an assortment of disorders. What many people in the U.S. don't know, however, is that the majority of patients in Germany obtain the herb not "like candy" but by prescription. It is also available over the counter, but people generally prefer using the prescription variety, both because it has been tested and proved to be effective through standardization, and also because it can then be reimbursed under that country's current health-care system.

Germany's government standards regarding over-the-counter

medicinal therapies is much less stringent than our own. Trial periods are shorter, and anecdotal information is considered acceptable support of a medicine's safety and efficacy.

The herb's ready availability both in Germany and here at home has its good aspects and its bad: It means more people have access to the medications they need and that if, after clinical diagnosis, people are unable to see a doctor for regular treatment, they have an option to do something to help themselves. Conversely, it also means that many people put themselves at risk, taking medications they shouldn't, in amounts that may not be safe, and sometimes for a condition they have self-diagnosed incorrectly.

So, in spite of its easy accessibility in Germany, where the herb's effects are government-recognized as therapeutic, doctors recommend that the herb be treated with the same caution as any chemical medication.

Is there anyone who shouldn't even try St. John's Wort?

Yes, some populations should bypass treatment on the herb for potent therapies that better treat their more serious disorders. These include the most severe cases of depression, such as melancholia and psychotic depression, as well as all cases of bipolar affective disorder. If you are having suicidal thoughts and have considered succumbing to them for even a moment, you need immediate treatment that St. John's Wort has not yet been proven to provide. See a doctor right away to explore antidepressant options.

Complicating illnesses that are concurrent with the depression disorder and require additional medication would indicate another form of therapy is needed, since the actions of St. John's Wort in relation to other drugs is yet unknown. Some recent cases suggest that those with a history of seizure disorders or stroke might be particularly wary, although links between these conditions and St. John's Wort have not been investigated and the cases may prove to be unrelated to herb use.

Side effects of St. John's Wort sometimes include nervousness, sleeplessness, and anxiety, so it could worsen bipolar and anxiety disorders. Anecdotal evidence supports these cautions, leaning heavily toward this simple conclusion: St. John's Wort has no positive effects on severe mental illness. If you have the severe symptoms, see your doctor.

I believe other populations may be at risk as well, such as childbearing women and those who are trying to become pregnant. The common belief of the medical community is that any substance with chemical effects should be avoided, even those that are plant-based, unless its impact on unborn fetuses and potential to promote birth defects (teratogenicity) has been discovered to be negligible. In addition, in one test on rodents, females displayed uterine contractions. Granted, these were rats, and the side effect has not been duplicated in human trials, but it is something of which a pregnant woman should be made aware. Nursing mothers should likewise use caution—many chemicals are easily passed to the infant through breast milk.

Since St. John's Wort has been shown to have some effect on estrogen levels, women with health conditions that are adversely affected by higher estrogen levels, such as some breast and uterine cancers, might want to use extra caution with this remedy. These cautions should all be balanced, however, with the recognition that no connection between harmful effects to fetuses or nursing infants or to women with estrogen-related illnesses have been noted in Germany, where it must be assumed that a number of women suffering from depression have used the drug during pregnancy and while breast-feeding. And that sometimes the risk is outweighed by other risk factors—such as the danger of the depression being left untreated. Examine your other treatment options. And if you and your doctor agree St. John's Wort is worth the risk, try to find extracts that do not use alcohol as their base. Still, I would urge caution and suggest the exploration of other, more conventional therapies.

Finally, people of certain ages may be more vulnerable to harsher side effects with herbal extracts, just as they are with synthetic drugs, such as the elderly and children. We simply do not know enough to be able to rule out risk. Talk with your pediatrician about the potential hazards and your other options. For the elderly, the dangers must be judged against another risk—25% of all suicides occur in the elderly population and many are the result of untreated depression. While St. John's Wort is not my treatment of choice for depressions that include suicidal ideation, talk with your doctor, family, and friends to try to get a more detached and balanced picture of your choices.

How come the government doesn't support more research into alternative therapies?

Actually, it is beginning to rally behind this "cause." In 1992, The Office of Alternative Medicine (OAM) was created as a division of the National Institutes of Health (NIH). NIH is itself one of eight health agencies under the aegis of the U.S. Public Health Service, and so falls under the administration of the U.S. Department of Health and Human Services (DHHS).

The NIH is the hub of the federal government's biomedical research initiatives and the leader in worldwide medical issues. Its focus on alternative medicine, as expressed through the formation of OAM, is a clear indication that these approaches will be taken more seriously.

OAM's charter is to aid in the dissemination of information and data analysis for "alternative medical treatment modalities." OAM also provides information to the public through a "clearinghouse," but does not offer referrals to alternative medical treatments or doctors who practice them. One indication of the government's new interest in alternative medicines is the budget for OAM, which has more than doubled in just five years, from just $2 million in 1992 to $12 million in 1997. Although this is still relatively "small potatoes" in terms of the funding needed to address alternative treatments for depression and the myriad of other disorders out there, it represents a huge jump, and reflects an increasing commitment to this area of research. With the money OAM will fund small-scale studies into a number of alternative therapies.

The National Cancer Institute, the largest of NIH's institutes, also dedicates money and support for research into alternative remedies (quite a bit of information about St. John's Wort comes through this agency), through its division for the study of natural products.

More and more, government agencies are coming around to support what has been called the "four Rs" for plant-based medicines: recognition, respectability, and reasonable regulation. That means medical organizations are joining patients in urging federal regulators to acknowledge the challenges that face alternative therapies like St. John's Wort in the marketplace. It supports the idea that more information needs to be made available both to patients and their caregivers.

Why hasn't St. John's Wort been approved as a depression medication in the U.S. yet? What's involved?

I've heard several people suggest that there is some sort of conspiracy, orchestrated by the medical establishment and pharmaceutical companies, behind the lack of federal approvals for herbal remedies. Actually, the vast majority of doctors would welcome any safe, effective method of treating depression with open arms, regardless of its origin. If we appear hesitant to throw the medical establishment's weight behind many botanicals, it is because we have witnessed so many fads come and go, as well as the toll they have taken on our patients in terms of crushed hopes, time wasted, and occasionally in outright dangerous effects. *Laetrile* comes to mind.

Before doctors jump on any kind of bandwagon, they (and I) want to be sure. We try to be sure—very sure. Despite its faults, the FDA's cautious approach has this as its governing principle: in the light of public demand for quick approvals, to be as certain as possible that people will not be hurt. The FDA might make some mistakes; but it is correct about literally hundreds more chemical-based medicines, i.e., these scientific failures that never made it to the shelves to hurt people.

As for the pharmaceutical industry's role in the suspected "conspiracy," the truth is simply that it is all about money. These companies are not typically out actively to crush new medical options like St. John's Wort, just to profit from them if they can. And if these companies see no profit margin, they simply aren't interested in "coughing up" the money to get the substance tested. So cost becomes the significant factor in the challenges facing herbal remedies in the U.S.

In order to become federally approved for treatment of a recognized disease or disorder in the U.S., a medicine must first meet the well-specified criteria of the Food and Drug Administration (FDA). These criteria involve rigorous, double-blind studies using established standards (i.e. recognized scales for rating depression before and after treatment), and require meticulously documented results. Years of work go into producing the clinical data supplied to the FDA, the results of clinical trials involving 2,000 to 4,000 patients. For a new antidepressant, three phases of research must lead to presentation of at least two large scale "pivotal" studies. The studies must be placebo-controlled and the new antidepressant must be significantly more effective (usually, at least a 20% difference in response rates). There must also be at least one year of longer term safety data, as well as a double-blind study of relapse prevention. The costs involved in such testing are astronomical—estimates put it anywhere between $35 and $200 million, depending on whom you ask. Expenses include sophisticated equipment, manufacture of highly standardized batches of the drug being tested, fees for patients and doctors, use of hospital facilities for monitoring patients, and the processing of the reams of data generated.

Who foots the bill? We all do to some extent in the prices we pay for brand-name products. Government grants support some such studies in one form or another, but the pharmaceutical companies are clearly the leading source of research on new medications. Why do they do it? Not for purely humanitarian reasons—profit is their main motive. Before the clinical trials begin, pharmaceutical companies apply for patents of the chemical formulas used in the testing, sometimes man-made versions of chemicals found naturally in botanicals. The company then "owns" the medicine or process for a time. If the therapy is successful and becomes approved, billions of dollars may be earned by the pharmaceutical company while the patent is valid. After that, generic versions of the drug can be made and sold by other companies, a competition that produces lower prices.

And that's where the problem facing herbal remedies comes in. Companies patent man-made formulas and mechanical or chemical processes, but no one can own the "right" to a plant. If a whole-herb form of St. John's Wort were tested and approved, anyone meeting FDA quality standards in processing and content would be able to manufacture and sell the herb-based medicine immediately. The company that sponsored such testing would be facing competition from other firms who would have benefited from its outlay of millions in research funds. In today's economy, it would take a very community-spirited CEO to make that kind of commitment without an exclusive right to the profits it would generate. Pharmaceutical companies—just like managed-care medical-insurance providers—look for a return on their investment in your health.

Still, there is some opportunity here for profit. In 1994, five patents were granted on botanically based medicinal products. That is the reason pharmaceutical companies are so interested in isolating the "marker" agent or agents in St. John's Wort responsible for its antidepressant effects (as well as its antiviral and cancer-fighting constituents). The mechanical process by which extracts or concentrations of active ingredients of St. John's Wort have yet to be assigned patients.

Some people feel the FDA's review process and its rigorous examination of effectiveness and safety data are unnecessary. Medical opponents of that view point to hundreds of substances that were proven dangerous during just such intensive scrutiny, even after a history of so-called "benign" treatment, such as diethylstilbestrol (DES), which was once used to prevent miscarriages but subsequently found to have negative effects on a fetus. Many stories like this exist to support a close examination of any substance being used for therapeutic reasons. We just need to balance caution with the realities of the obstacles facing an herbal remedy in a somewhat hostile financial climate.

Some good news for St. John's Wort: Recently, the FDA appointed a new director, who has moved toward a shorter review period for substances being submitted for approval. It used to take an average of thirty-two months for a drug to pass through the FDA approval process; now the wait is just fifteen months. That has had a big impact on numbers of drugs receiving approval. In 1986 only twenty were approved; in 1996 that number more than doubled, soaring to fifty-three. In addition, drug manufacturers are now required to pay a fee when they submit new substances for approval; this is imposed to help pay for the expenses of reviews, and will help support "orphan drugs," which do not receive such powerful financial support.

What's happening with the major U.S. study I've heard rumors about?

The study has begun! Under the auspices of the National Institute for Mental Health, what many believe will be a definitive clinical trial on St. John's Wort's effects on mild to moderate depression is now under way in the U.S. NIMH has dedicated over $4 million to the study, which is being coordinated by Jonathan Davidson, MD, at its coordinating site, Duke University Medical Center, in Durham, North Carolina. The study will also involve patients in approximately ten satellite sites around the country. Altogether, more than 300 patients will be enrolled and monitored in what's being called a "three-arm, double-blind clinical efficacy study." In simpler terms, that means the study will be assessing the effects of three substances—900 milligrams per day of standardized *Hypericum* extract (also known as St. John's Wort); 50 milligrams per day of one of the most successful and popular of the newer SSRI antidepressants, sertraline (Zoloft); and a placebo. It also means that no one participating in the study will know until conclusion of the acute phase just who got what, not even the physicians working directly with the patients.

The study is intended to address many of the concerns our own medical establishment continues to have with European studies: standardization of doses; uniform criteria for patients (using a recognized scale to define the patients' levels of depression and relief); long-term monitoring for side effects and relapse (although the "acute" phase of the trial lasts only 8 weeks, patients who demonstrate improvement on the herb will be monitored in follow-up visits for an additional four months); and the possibility of a placebo effect that diminishes with time.

As of this writing the study was still seeking a pharmaceutical supplier for the materials to be used in the study. In a double-blind trial such as this, all three pills—the placebo, SSRI, and St. John's Wort—must look, smell, and taste identical to one another and yet be coded in such a way that while no one will have a clue which is being administered, data may be accurately compiled at trial's end. That's a hefty investment in and of itself: an estimated 309,852 pills will be required altogether.

Patient recruitment was scheduled to begin June 1998. Enrollment will take some time, as patients are screened and rated on scales of depression, checked for overall health, and evaluated for their potential as test subjects—to reach the intended number of 336 individuals with depression disorder.

Patients who have depression diagnosed as severe, those who are suicidal, hospitalized patients, and people who have used the herbal remedy before but experienced unpleasant side effects will be eliminated from the study. If you are interested in participating and enrollment is still open, you and your doctor can find out more by calling or writing to Dr. Davidson at the center:

Duke University Medical Center
Durham, NC 27710
(919) 684-8111

The trial's active phase with the subjects will last six months in total. But the follow-up period, when the data from 336 cases is being compiled and analyzed, will take many months more. It could be as long as three years from the start of the clinical trials before the final conclusions are announced.

Is all this about going through the motions? Doesn't everyone in these agencies really think St. John's Wort is okay to use now?

If everyone was one hundred percent sure, St. John's Wort would already be approved. There are still lurking questions, however, so neither the National Institute of Mental Health nor the FDA considers it "safe" to use on depression right now. Both organizations urge caution. I agree that care should be exercised until we find out more. My patients are using St. John's Wort under supervision of a doctor, and that's the best way to use *any* new therapy, most especially one that is still experimental. Consider that as you decide if St. John's Wort is the safest and most effective therapy for you.

FIVE

❦

Using St. John's Wort
As an Antidepressant:
What You Need to Know

*The Kim who came for her twenty-first visit with her
doctor wasn't the same woman who had walked through
the door for her first session. That Kim had been hollow-
eyed, with a kind of quiet desperation. Her smile was
actually a slightly scary grimace unsuccessfully attempting to disguise a constant inner fear and despair. That
Kim had seen an obstacle in every challenge, political
undercurrents in every personal contact, and a threat in
every change. Kim had suffered from mild depression
for years without truly acknowledging it, despite a clear
family history of the disorder. Her moods had ebbed and
flowed, with "down-times," as she put it, usually centered around the loss of a boyfriend or some unsettling
change at work. And then her mother became ill. For
nearly a year, Kim spent vacations shuttling long-
distance between her own apartment and her mother's
nursing home. The last straw fell when her mother's
death coincided with yet another career shift. It was all
too much. Kim's friends told an even bleaker story,
about a woman who had seemed to slowly lose all focus
and interest in her job, social life, and hobbies. Even
Kim was realizing that her inability to make decisions*

*was going to lead to some sort of dramatic confrontation
very soon—fear of that was simply making matters
worse. Kim was in the throes of one wicked episode of
major depression, of moderate to severe intensity. The
idea of St. John's Wort didn't even enter her doctor's
mind then. Kim began treatment with one of the newer
SSRIs. The first one had side effects that made contin-
uance intolerable, so another was prescribed. The second also had similar side effects—uncomfortable, but
tolerable. Kim noticed a change within just three weeks.
The drug was slowly but surely pulling her out of the
depths, so she chose to remain on the treatment. Kim's
depression was in remission seven months after she began her visits. But she had no intention of prolonging
maintenance therapy on the antidepressant, fearing continued side effects just as she was feeling well, even on
a lowered dose. Her doctor suggested a combination of
alternatives, which involved cognitive behavioral therapy to help her strengthen coping skills, regular exercise, and St. John's Wort. Kim agreed and the
antidepressant was withdrawn slowly. After discontinu-
ation of the medication, Kim has remained symptom-free
for five months.*

You learned the results of the clinical studies. Listened to
the media reports. You checked the worldwide web to see
what sufferers were saying about their experiences with St.
John's Wort. Now is the time to make the decision: Do I use
it myself? How?

There is no question that interest in herbal remedies is on
the rise. Terms are being coined for them—phytomedicines,
nutraceuticals and international symposia and medical con-
gresses are being held to exchange information about them
across the medical and herbalist communities.

How come people choose alternative therapies like St. John's Wort if conventional treatments work so well?

Negative images persist about the use of drugs for any kind
of illness, and particularly mental illness, about which negative
myths abound already. This fear, born largely of false beliefs,
prevents many from getting the help they can from conven-

tional drug therapy. Then again, many people choose alternative therapies for treatment because they don't know much about the other options that exist. Many simply aren't aware of the incredibly wide range of medications available to treat their disorder, or that newer varieties have significantly fewer side effects than any depression medicine encountered before.

Some people turn to alternative therapies only when more conventional treatments fail. While antidepressants, psychotherapy, or some combination of the two are ultimately successful in approximately 80% of all cases of depression, that figure still leaves many people unaccounted for. In addition, significant numbers of those helped by antidepressants eventually discontinue therapy because of side effects. Among the most annoying long-term side effects of antidepressants are sexual dysfunction, especially difficulty reaching orgasm, and weight gain. Many who aren't helped by medication respond to electroconvulsive therapy (ECT). It is a fact, however, that the potential to relapse after effective ECT is high. Moreover, while clearly a valuable treatment, some people experience significant memory difficulties (usually reversible within several months) and ECT remains one of our most stigmatized and misunderstood therapies.

Cost is a factor some people mention when asked why they have made the switch to alternative treatments. Managed care has made periodic doctor visits and prescriptions an option for some, but has restricted benefits and access to care for others. Depending upon your employer's health insurance plan, your conventional therapy might be covered in full, covered for only a short time (the period of acute treatment only), or not at all. The risk of relapse if treatment is not continued is high for people with more chronic or recurrent depressions. And, sadly, some people remain uninsured for health coverage. The $100 a month on average spent for treatment with some antidepressants may not even be a possibility for these depression sufferers.

For other people, treatment choices revolve around the issue of trust, preference, and control. Recent surveys have shown this is often the case with highly educated patients, who increasingly wish to take control of their treatment into their own hands if at all possible. People like this might make more of an effort to stay informed of news, including medical breakthroughs. They tend to be more skeptical of authority and less willing to put "blind" trust in a physician. Such folks have found that control is easier to achieve with an herbal treatment than a prescription drug which requires regular interaction with a busy doctor who, depending on the level of communication skills, may not be involving patients as much as they like. For many, it is simply a dislike of using any "drug," i.e., a chemical synthesized by a pharmaceutical company and prescribed by a licensed physician, however safe and effective it has proven in the long term. Perhaps it is a lack of trust for the "pharmaceutical-medical complex," or a sense that a large profit should not be made from the relief of others' suffering that motivates some toward alternate therapies. Beliefs that "natural is better" and holistic views about health and nature are often common. St. John's Wort appeals to this wide-ranging group of people.

Whatever their reasons, increasingly, patients are turning their attention to St. John's Wort. Conventional medical practitioners are responding to the rise in interest, too. More than half of all family physicians surveyed in a recent poll routinely suggest alternative therapy to their patients or use some form of it themselves. The American Medical Association passed a resolution not long ago encouraging its members to become "better informed regarding alternative medicine," and went on to recommend that doctors actively participate in studies on these treatments. Furthermore, courses in alternative medicine are being added in medical schools recognized as leaders in the field—over a third of them now offer such instruction. Since a lack of basic knowledge or even awareness of these alternatives has been responsible for many doctors' lack of support for such treatments, this is a significant step forward. More schools are bound to follow the example set by institutions like the Harvard Medical School and Johns Hopkins.

I don't know . . . I just don't trust any medicines that come from plants. Give me science every time.

Actually, medical science has nearly always found its inspiration in plants. You've probably used aspirin at one time or another—it is the classic example of a synthetic drug made from a chemical (salicin) first discovered in the bark of willows and plants of the spirea genus. Digitalis, a powerful cardiac stimulant used in the treatment of heart conditions, was "discovered" because of centuries of anecdotal treatment with foxglove, the plant whose marker agent this chemical mimics. Many antibiotics' ancestors are isolations of chemicals first noted in plant remedies, as are some cancer-fighting agents, quinine, morphine, and the first synthetic drug used to treat psychosis, reserpine. And, of course, lithium carbonate, one of the first-line treatments for manic depression, is a natural salt of the lithium ion—a chemical right out of the periodic table of elements.

Why has St. John's Wort suddenly become so "hot" as an alternative antidepressant?

There are a number of reasons behind the herb's present "hot" status: Alternative remedies on the whole got a boost in 1992 when the government agency known as the Office of Alternative Medicine, or OAM, was initiated through congressional mandate, and again in 1994 when Congress passed the Dietary Supplement Health and Education Act (DSHEA). The act lifted many of the restrictions governing products like herbal remedies, including how they could be labeled and promoted. Under the new act, companies that make dietary supplements (also called nutritional supplements) continue to be free from the necessity of submitting proof that their products are therapeutically effective. Further, whereas before such products couldn't make a health-related claim of *any* kind, now they may *suggest* treatment applications by describing what body functions the products might enhance as long as they make no direct claims to treat a medical illness. The Food and Drug Administration probably will not let this matter stand, as is, for long. So, for the time being, while no package of St. John's Wort should say it can be used to treat depression, the manufacturer can now openly claim to "improve mood." That seems like a pretty fine line to many in the medical field—one with the potential to confuse and mislead consumers. It is one which a number of unscrupulous companies routinely tiptoe along and occasionally even cross. And, as St. John's Wort consumers are often doctors' patients, many physicians have been concerned about the possibility of false "pseudo-medical" claims. In any case, the 1994 enactment of the new law opened the door for many botanical-based products, like St. John's Wort, which followed.

The same year the DSHEA arrived, the *Journal of Geriatric Psychiatry and Neurology* published an issue with seventeen separate studies on the herb. Just over a year later, on August 3, 1996, the *British Medical Journal* published a scholarly analysis of some of those same studies, plus many more. In all, twenty-three studies were reviewed, involving 1,757 patients and covering a range of the herb's various effects—antidepressant, antiviral, and cancer-fighting (antineoplastic). The conventional medical world took notice. Awareness of the herb had already permeated the World Wide Web, with discussions on St. John's Wort popping up in newsgroups all over the Internet, creating enormous word of mouth "buzz" about the herb. Companies producing the herbal remedy also began utilizing this instant source of information, posting sites for a not-always-accurate source of information on an international scale.

Hard on the heels of that *BMJ* report came the first consumer book on the subject of St. John's Wort published in America. The information it presented arrived at a time when interest in alternatives was increasing. The media, hungry for stories on this subject to feed a growing consumer interest, leapt on the story. An avalanche of press attention followed, in particular a report by the television news magazine *20/20* and a number of articles in respected popular publications such as *Newsweek* and the *Washington Post*. St. John's Wort had already been making a regular appearance for years in herbal newsletters and in consumer magazines with a focus on health, like *HerbalGram* and *Prevention* magazine.

Since cost is such a factor in choosing alternative therapies, how much is treatment with St. John's Wort?

A month-long supply of St. John's Wort tablets typically runs in the neighborhood of twenty dollars. There are some brands selling for as high as twenty-seven and others on sale for as low as fifteen dollars. Liquid extracts, which some herbalists believe are more potent, tend to run a little higher. (Clinical trials tend to use the liquid extract or tablets made from such extracts.) Teas have not been the focus of any clinical trials, although anecdotal reports indicate they are nowhere near as concentrated or effective.

Compare that average $20-per-month expense to the cost of a similar period's therapy with a prescription medication. Because there are so many drug options, prices range quite a bit, with generic forms of most of the tricyclics being cheaper. Most of the newer medications, such as the SSRIs, cost at least $60–$80 per month. However, if your dosage is very high or your doctor is prescribing the medication in a less efficient way (i.e., two 75-mg Effexor® tablets rather than one 150-mg tablet), the costs can be double or even triple $60 per month. Prozac and Remeron will be the first to go off patent, so they may be the first available in a generic form.

I hate the idea of drugs or psychotherapy. Why shouldn't I just go straight to St. John's Wort?

I regret sounding like a broken record, but you should never reach a diagnosis and develop a treatment plan for anything as complex as depression without first consulting with a physician. If you've already done that and learned that your mood disorder is not too severe (i.e., you're not actively suicidal and you're able to work and function okay at home), then there is no real reason you shouldn't ask your doctor about this herbal remedy. If St. John's Wort doesn't work, though, you should talk about your dislike of drugs and other therapies with your doctor. Maybe more information about the conventional treatments may help you to give a standard medication a "trial run." Incidentally, I make the same recommendation for people who would rather be treated with psychotherapy alone, instead of medication. If you've not noticed an honestly significant difference after six weeks of St. John's Wort therapy, it's probably not the right treatment for you.

Everyone talks about how St. John's Wort "works" on depression's symptoms. Forget the science—I want to know how I'll *feel*.

One of the issues American researchers have with many of the European studies is that the degree and nature of the relief experienced while on St. John's Wort is not spelled out in criteria that can be reliably measured and compared. If therapy is successful, the European studies suggest that a few "feelings" consistently emerge:

- St. John's Wort has been shown to lessen the classic feelings of depression—the low moods, dejection, sense of worthlessness and hopelessness that are common hallmarks of this mood disorder.
- Anxiety might be lessened—overall, an evening out of extremes, to create a more "normal" emotional response to life.
- Quality of sleep appears to improve as well, although only in one very specific way—St. John's Wort doesn't help you get to sleep, but when you do slumber, it may enhance the quality of your sleep.
- Some patients have remarked that their appetites return to more normal levels; the lack of interest in food so typical of depression lessens and you may again have gusto for food.

In more intimate terms, here is how some patients have described their positive reactions to St. John's Wort:

- "Wonderful, almost giddy."
- "Just as good as, if not better than, the antidepressants I used to take—and at least I'm not losing sexual function or my hair."
- "Suddenly, I'm interested in life again."
- "I'd forgotten what it felt like to be normal."
- "It was like a dark cloud lifted."

My friend says St. John's Wort is a placebo—it just makes you *think* you feel better.

This is actually a more complex statement than it may appear. To settle this question about any therapeutic substance with a degree of accuracy, you need to test the treatment in what researchers call a double-blind clinical trial, which uses a procedure for disguising and distributing the medications to prevent *both* patients and doctors from knowing just who is getting what. In the case of St. John's Wort studies comparing the herbal remedy's effects to those of conventional antidepressants, that would mean that it's not known who's being treated with the herb or the synthetic antidepressant. When double-blind controls are not in place, you can never be sure if a patient's response is an accurate representation of what the medication is doing, or if patients were simply experiencing the symptoms and reactions they *thought* matched the medicine. Even in a single-blind study, where doctors are aware of who has received the placebo and who's gotten the medicine, a doctor might inadvertently signal to patients what therapy they're on through a careless question or significant glance. That's why double-blinds are considered the best way to conduct such experimentation. Certainly, about 20% to 40% of people in any given study will have a placebo response even to a genuine therapy, but the overall rates of such a response should be approximately the same for St. John's Wort and the standard medication, and thus cancel each other out. The best controlled studies use random assignment (people can't pick which treatment they receive), double-blind medication, and rating response with an accurate scale, especially if the rating is done by a trained observer who has not been part of your regular treatment. In an "ideal" study, both the new treatment (e.g., St. John's Wort) and the standard treatment (e.g., Zoloft®) would be significantly better than a placebo. Typically, this would mean that St. John's Wort and the standard control work at least 60% of the time, with placebo helping less than 40% of the participants.

Many European studies of St. John's Wort did not use double-blind trials. But some have a scientific basis, albeit an imperfect one, for the medical world's hoopla over St. John's Wort. The results of those studies demonstrated a noticeably better response to St. John's Wort than to placebo. In fact, in trials using a standard antidepressant results for St. John's Wort have been close to those on the conventional medication. A well-designed clinical trial currently being conducted in the U.S. will utilize the double-blind approach to compare placebo, St. John's Wort, and Zoloft®.

Interestingly, research has shown that more severe depressions tend to respond much better to antidepressants than placebo, whereas the differences are often smaller with milder cases of the disorder. Does this mean that mild depression isn't a true disorder? No! That mild depression is purely emotional or psychological and not the result of biochemical changes?

No! Does that mean St. John's Wort is just a placebo, because it works best on mild conditions, where placebos have a strong effect? No! It probably just indicates that milder depressions are more likely to end quicker and that it's harder to show a drug-placebo difference. If St. John's Wort consistently outperforms placebo in mild depression, it's more than just a placebo! And it could be that St. John's Wort's unknown antidepressant ingredients do not alleviate those specific chemical reactions that are found in the disorder's more severe presentations.

If no one is sure hypericin is the ingredient that works on depression after all, why should I use a standardized extract?

It's true that extracts are currently standardized to ensure the amount of hypericin relative to the other contents of the remedy. And, yes, hypericin may not be the chemical responsible for the herb's primary actions in depression. Still, while we may not know exactly what is happening, we *do* know from the results of many studies that using hypericin as the yardstick for measuring standardization is a valid way of ensuring an extract's overall effectiveness in battling depression. It may be that hypericin will turn out to be the major active constituent after all, or simply that when you concentrate and measure hypericin, it is taking other important agents "along for the ride." In this sense, hypericin could continue to be the herb's marker for the active ingredient(s), a standard by which we measure the herb's contents, until we learn what's principally responsible for its various actions.

I am about to begin treating my depression with St. John's Wort but heard that if you take it and eat certain foods, it could kill you. Should I be watching what I eat?

These fears arose from the long-held belief that something in the herb acted as a potent inhibitor of monoamine oxidase. Inhibition of MAO results in an increase in the amounts of chemicals in your body that are normally broken down by the MAO enzyme. One such chemical, tyramine, is found in many common aged foods, such as cheese and sour cream, as well as Italian (fava) broad beans, beer, and overripe banana peels. Multiplying already MAOI-increased levels with the additional supply of tyramine introduced by these foods could, theoretically, increase the risk of producing a dangerously steep rise in blood pressure.

Subsequent testing has revealed that hypericin is most likely not the MAO inhibitor researchers once thought, at least in liquid extracts of the herb, and that St. John's Wort may not have a clinically significant effect on MAO enzyme activity. Further, if such an interaction *were* a risk for St. John's Wort, we should be seeing hundreds of toxic responses in Germany, where St. John's Wort has been used by millions of people for over a decade. That is simply not happening. No one is known to have died from the interaction of St. John's Wort and certain foods. A single suspicious instance of a woman suffering stroke caused by high blood pressure while on St. John's Wort therapy has recently surfaced. There are suspicions that an adulterated dose of the herb was used or some MAOI-potent whole-herb form of the herbal remedy. It has been noted that the studies demonstrating little MAOI activity and low impact by hypericin were conducted on liquid extracts—the whole-herb forms of the herb have not been a adequately tested for these effects.

So, until all doubt surrounding St. John's Wort MAOI action has been eliminated, you should stick to using liquid-extract-based forms of the herb (many tablets are derived from such extracts) and perhaps cut down on or eliminate these foods:

FOODS CONTAINING TYRAMINE

aspartame (a sugar substitute)
red wine
beer and colored alcohols
aged cheeses (cheddar, colby, Camembert, Roquefort, Brie, Gruyère, mozzarella, Parmesan, Romano, blue provolone, Gouda, and Stilton
beans (broad fava, garbanzo, Italian, lentil, lima, navy, pinto, string beans, and snow peas)
sourdough and cheese breads or yeast breads served warm
preserved meats

　overripe or dried fruits (black bananas, raisins, figs, and
　　mincemeat mixtures)
　chocolate or cocoa
　monosodium glutamate, aka hydrolyzed vegetable pro-
　　tein, hydrolyzed plant protein (MSG, MVG, MPP)

There are more foods to avoid when on treatments with
MAOIs, as well as other medications, including over-the-
counter cold and flu medications, hay-fever remedies, decon-
gestants, nasal inhalants, asthma inhalants, diet pills,
amphetamines, narcotics, as well as the herbs yohimbe, licorice root, and *Ephedra* (also called Ma Huang). Ask your doctor for a complete list of substances to eliminate on an MAOI
therapy.

My feeling is that eating these foods while taking normal
doses of St. John's Wort should not make you ill. But be alert
when you eat them while on the therapy—monitor your side
effects more carefully for a time after you have combined such
foods and the remedy, and see your doctor at the first hint of
any serious effects.

Can I drink alcohol at all when I'm taking St. John's Wort?

St. John's Wort actually has been used to flavor alcoholic
beverages such as brandies in the past, but those flavorings
used extracts that were free of hypericin. The chemical was
removed not through concern over its interaction with alcohol, but because of a scare resulting from St. John's Wort's
suspected tie to photosensitization. However, my take is that
if you are using an herbal remedy instead of a medication,
you should treat it like one and there is no medication that
is truly safe to take with alcohol. If you can't avoid alcohol,
limit your intake to the same cautious levels you would if
you were on a prescription drug. Remember, too, that beer
and many alcoholic beverages, like red wine, contain tyramine, a chemical that is released by MAOI medications and
which may also be produced by the actions of St. John's
Wort. (The jury is still out on that one.) Even more importantly, people who are depressed should not drink because it
can lower mood or increase suicidal ideations or tendencies.

I heard reactions to antidepressant drugs could be toxic. How careful should I be?

You should be very careful, just as you would mixing any two drugs. I reiterate—if you are using St. John's Wort as a treatment for a specific disorder or disease, you are using it as a medication. This is an area that has gotten little attention in European studies. In tests on rodents, St. John's Wort was observed in relation to several specific drugs: in those studies, the herb seems to interact poorly with dopamine-reducing agents such as Haloperidol, which tend to block the herb's effects; reserpine action may be blocked by use of St. John's Wort, so those two substances should not be used in tandem either. Some narcotics will induce even stronger deep-sleep responses when St. John's Wort is also being administered. The questions concerning MAO activity by the herb have been addressed earlier and combined use with the MAOI class of antidepressants should not occur.

The issue of drug interactions will have to be investigated as the herb is examined for FDA approval. Safety in use with other medications is not necessary to win approval—virtually every medication has known interactions—but before St. John's Wort is recommended specific problems would have to be identified. As it stands now, since we are still so uncertain about the herb's effects, no doctor can say with certainty the herb won't cause a harmful reaction, or nullify the effects of your other chemical therapies. (If you are using an antidepressant and want to explore options to augment that treatment, see the list of alternative therapies listed in Chapter 9 that will not precipitate a chemical interaction.)

How could St. John's Wort therapy interact with recreational drugs?

Not well, I'm sure. Such drugs often reverse or otherwise interfere with the actions of therapeutic substances. Cocaine and other diet pills could be particularly toxic. My suggestion is to discuss your use of recreational drugs with your physician, to learn their possible effects on your health (illegal substances often contribute to feelings of depression), to examine whether you are using them to suppress symptoms of your mood disorder (this could only work temporarily and may adversely affect more long-term help), and to determine if you are using them addictively. If so, you need to address the addiction before you can begin to focus on the depression.

Cold and flu season is rolling around. Can I take St. John's Wort while I'm on an over-the-counter cold medication?

This is not an interaction that has been examined in any clinical test. I'm sure that through the years in Germany and elsewhere in Europe, people have doubled up on medications this way with no dire effects, but I wouldn't recommend trying it. Not enough is known about what happens when St. John's Wort is exposed to other such substances in your system. Some commercial cold remedies and antihistamines contain ingredients that are enhanced by the use of MAOI antidepressants. We're still not sure what kind of MAOI effect some forms of St. John's Wort are capable of, so it would be wise to check labels carefully or generally steer clear of *any* interactions. In the event you get a cold or the flu, ask yourself: Which set of symptoms will it be easier to live with for a time—the ones accompanying the cold or depression? Decide which you can afford to ignore or treat with nondrug therapies until the doubling of disorders has passed.

I already take a few herbal remedies. They work great for me. Would I have to stop taking them if I go on St. John's Wort?

I would also avoid using this herbal remedy at the same time you are using other botanical products. Not enough is known about St. John's Wort's interaction with other herbs to ensure an uncomplicated mixing of such substances. Even herbalists frown on an *ad lib* mixing of herbs. Instead, stick to one herb at a time, using the one that addresses your most pernicious complaint. When that has been eliminated target another. If you must address more than one at a time, do your homework and find an herbal remedy that targets the most symptoms and conditions. See the resource chapter for a few good herbal references that can help guide you.

How much St. John's Wort should I take? How often?

When consuming commercial preparations of the herb, I always recommend following dosing directions. If a range of doses are suggested, begin with the lowest one indicated. Don't worry that it will be "weak"—in prescription antidepressant therapy we often find that some people respond to low doses just as well as the higher ones. Low doses certainly produce far fewer serious side effects.

Different brands use a variety of ratios of whole herb to standardized hypericin content. In the overview of twenty-three studies so often used as a benchmark for use of St. John's Wort, 300–900 milligrams of the whole herb seemed the most effective dose, but no study has really focused on the crucial issue of minimum dosing, or what effect varying levels may have on the diverse mood-disorder symptoms.

Here is one formula used to determine dose in most clinical trials, using the measurements for raw herb and hypericin most commonly found in standardized extracts (although different ratios exist, you should always end up with the same approximate dose of 1 mg of hypericin daily):

Amount of raw herb . . .	**300 mg**	**450 mg**
Containing this amount of standardized hypericin . . .	**0.3%**	**0.2%**
Taken between 1 and 3 times a day (feelings are mixed on the best dose; start low)		
To reach a total of . . .	300 mg raw herb and 90 micrograms (approx. 1 mg) hypericin at low dose;	450 mg raw herb and 90 micrograms (approx. 1 mg) hypericin at low dose;
	OR	OR
	900 mg raw herb and 270 micrograms (approx. 2.7 mg) hypericin at high dose	1350 mg raw herb and 270 micrograms (approx. 2.7 mg) hypericin at high dose

*To determine total
  amount of hypericin
  taken daily,
  multiply...*   **300 × 0.3**   **450 × 0.2**

Generally, if on a high dose, people divide it into three, spaced regularly throughout the day. If you are using St. John's Wort to treat depression-related sleeping disturbances, the final dose should be taken with a snack before bedtime.

Here's how dosing typically breaks down for the herb's various forms, in case dosing suggestions are not provided (not a good sign):

- By weight, 2–4 grams of the dried herb is indicated (again, start low, shift upward only if necessary)
- A liquid extract using the ratio of 1:1 (one part herb in grams to one part solvent in milliliters) in 25% alcohol would be dosed at between 2 and 4 milliliters (.2–1.0 mg), anywhere from 5–15 is typical, but don't be surprised if some brands list higher numbers—just begin with the lowest dose suggested
- A tincture using the ratio of 1:10 in 45% alcohol would be dosed at between 2 and 4 milliliters ($^1/_4$–1 teaspoon). (**Note**: This amount of alcohol is not a problem.)
- An infusion (tea) is taken three times daily in small cups (not recommended)
- In powdered form, 2–4 grams of the whole herb (0.2–1.0 grams of hypericin) has been suggested
  (See more on dosing with homegrown remedies in Chapter Eight.)

When using homegrown remedies, dosing is harder to determine, as the concentration of active agents might be far less or more than levels found in standardized commercial preparations. There are many, many chemical agents at play in a whole plant. Their unique interaction in a species, even within an individual stem, is almost impossible to predict. Growing conditions, strength of genetic strain, and environmental situation all combine to make each crop a new mystery. Add to that the variables different qualities of processing bring to the mix and you are left with a big question mark. (See Chapter Eight on homegrown remedies.)

If you feel strongly about using nonstandardized sources of St. John's Wort be aware that you won't know how much of any single element you're getting. Now, many herbalists see this as a benefit of herbal dosing. They feel that the complex interplay between these elements is what makes an herb effective. Perhaps the active chemicals are more potent when supported by other constituents in the herb, or their side effects are lessened or alleviated by another agent. For that reason some people might prefer using willow bark over aspirin. That may be, or it may account for why a single herb may have a dozen or more suspected actions. Still, it cannot be ignored that clinical studies consistently reproducing antidepressant effects have successfully used hypericin content as their marker for effective dosing.

Should I take my daily dose of St. John's Wort with food?

Nothing so far suggests that St. John's Wort works better on an empty stomach, so I recommend taking it with food for convenience. Consuming therapeutic medicines with a meal sometimes reduces the chance of nausea and stomach pain, both potential side effects from the use of St. John's Wort therapy.

How can I know how much hypericin is in a "standardized" dose?

The only way you can know is if the manufacturer tells you. Look for information provided on the packaging or label. Hopefully, the manufacturer has adhered to recent guidelines, which suggest a set of specific tests to analyze and ensure standardized levels of chemical agents in herb extracts. The three recommended for *Hypericum* include:

- a spectrophotometric-analysis procedure
- thin layer chromatography (TLC)
- high-performance liquid chromatography (HPLC)

Do those names need to mean anything to you? Probably not; but you should know that a combination of all three sophisticated techniques have been suggested for *Hypericum* (more than for many other substances standardized in this way), because the nature of the herb's active constituents is still unknown. Scientists want to be sure they've got everything in there.

How long before it starts to work? And when should I stop taking it?

The antidepressive effects of therapy with St. John's Wort are typically not expected until at least 10–14 days of treatment, and in many cases do not become evident for as many as six weeks of treatment. If, however, you haven't experienced a noticeable alleviation of depressive symptoms—if you don't simply "feel better"—after six weeks, you should re-examine your therapy on the herb. Are you using a reputable brand, standardized to contain a certain level of active agents? Are you using the recommended dose? Have you been regular in your dosing, or did you miss several days? If you have done everything right, and the treatment still doesn't work, then stop using it. Don't waste more time than you have to on a therapy that fails you.

As for how long you should remain on St. John's Wort therapy, you should know that most clinical studies of St. John's Wort's effects tracked patients for no longer than 8 weeks, often less. Currently, no long-term studies exist that answer this question definitively. The anecdotal evidence runs the gamut of periods of duration and effectiveness, but I know of a number of patients on the herb who claim they experienced a noticeable drop in the herbal remedy's effectiveness over time. For some this came quickly, after just a few months of therapy (most likely they were simply experiencing a prolonged placebo response in that case); for others effects have lasted decades. Very few patients have been tracked, even informally, for long-term effectiveness, and the herb has been popular such a short time in the U.S. our own anecdotal evidence is not yet old enough to give us any real sense of when to stop. So my advice is simply to stay alert and consider intermittent dosing: stop using the herb when symptoms have disappeared for six months and start again only if they reappear. Until more is known about the herb, this seems the safest route. In the meantime, it is a matter of measuring your own personal risk-to-benefit ratio: Is how you're feeling right now worth any potential risks? Monitor your symptoms and side effects even more carefully as time passes. How is St. John's Wort working for *you*? When do *you* feel it has run its course?

Should I experiment with different dosages?

Consider a higher dose only if you started on a low dose and have not seen an effect. If, however, you began your therapy with the recommended dosage, I wouldn't fool around. The potential for experiencing side effects or more extreme side effects increases significantly as you increase your dose of *any* medication, and the same is true of herbal remedies. Also, keep in mind that there is little evidence that doses above 900 mg a day are effective.

What if I've missed a dose? Okay ... a few doses?

Just how many is "a few"? Neglecting to take your regular dose for a day or two probably would not affect your therapy. However, missing more than that could cause a dip in the plant's effectiveness. St. John's Wort's effects are completely reversible. Although St. John's Wort builds up to a small degree—hence the 2–6 weeks before you begin to see results—your body quickly rids itself of the herb after dosing has ceased. In scientific terms, that means a chemical agent has a very short elimination half-life, the period of time necessary for half the substance to be broken down and eliminated by your body. This particular herb's constituents don't linger in your system for very long (the half-life of hypericin has been estimated as low as twenty-five hours), so when you stop taking it, the effect established by regular use is soon lost, and the therapy stops having an effect. If you've missed more than a couple of doses, you may have to build up levels of St. John's Wort again over a number of weeks.

However, before you begin the cycle all over again, ask yourself: How serious am I about this therapy? If you are using St. John's Wort in the same fashion you would a drug—that is, not simply to "enhance" your mood but to seriously treat depression's symptoms—then you need to commit yourself to the routine of taking consistent doses of the herb at regular intervals. If you find you are repeatedly missing a dose, then that might signal a lack of interest or dedication to this therapy. Talk to your doctor and be honest about your situation.

Together, you might take a look at other therapies that interest you more or would suffer less from inattention.

I'd like to stop taking a tricyclic for my anxiety attacks. Will St. John's Wort adequately control my anxiety?

It is a question of severity, as is so often the case with St. John's Wort therapy. If you are experiencing feelings of nervous tension accompanying depression, or anxiety attacks that despite their disturbing nature are mild and not disruptive to your life, St. John's Wort may be an option for you. A few of the European studies have mentioned improvement of anxiety levels and alleviation of "nervous excitement particularly associated with menopause" for patients on the herb. It is difficult to tell from the haphazard methodology of many of these tests, however, if a true case of anxiety disorder was affected, or just the low levels of nervous tension sometimes felt by a person in an episode of major depression. If you were already considering stopping your tricyclic therapy, talk to your doctor about trying St. John's Wort. If she is amenable, perhaps you could give the herb a six-week trial. No promises can be made about whether it will be an adequate treatment of your particular manifestation of anxiety disorder, however. Even if further, more anxiety-targeted testing reveals an effect on that mood disturbance, no two people will react the same. Body chemistry comes into play, as do overall mental and physical health, environment, and social interaction. Exposure to stressors plays such an important role in anxiety disorders that it can not be discounted, either.

Will I have to keep taking St. John's Wort forever?

There are some "converts" in Germany who have been on the herb for a decade or more, with no buildup of side effects. But I have also heard reports of people complaining because its antidepressant effects seem to wear off after a year or so. If you do not have a history of chronic or recurrent depression, my advice would be to taper off the herb after you have been symptom-free for six months (the same period recommended for antidepressant-drug continuation-phase therapy, in order to prevent relapse of the acute episode). If your depression returns with a bang, begin treatment again. If not, use the herb at the first sign of an episode in the future.

I've been on Prozac for my depression and feel much better. Should I replace it with St. John's Wort? What's the best way to switch?

If you're happy with your current treatment, why switch? If it's just because there's currently so much "buzz" about the herb, it is probably not worth the risk. If cost or some other major factor is at play, however, you should first weigh it against the possibility that if you switch, there is no guarantee the St. John's Wort therapy will even work. What impact will months spent on a failed experiment with the herb take on your health and psyche? Is it worth switching after all?

If you do decide to switch, I would opt for the same "washout" period you would use between treatments of two synthetic drugs. Give your system time to rid itself of the Prozac before starting on the St. John's Wort—you reduce the risk of side effects from interactions and also reduce confusion over which remedy is having an effect. I'd suggest at least four to six weeks if possible. Talk to your doctor about the optimum period of time to wait between therapies.

I've been on St. John's Wort for six weeks but have seen no change whatsoever. How long should I wait?

The time frame for seeing results from St. John's Wort therapy ranges, but the average reaction time is 4–6 weeks, slightly longer than that of most antidepressants. If you have been using the herbal remedy for six weeks without an effect, are using a low dose, and can afford some more time on experimentation, try raising the dose slightly. If that is not the situation, however, don't waste another week. Stop the therapy and talk to your doctor about your other options.

Will St. John's Wort alone do the job?

If you routinely struggle with a restrained case of seasonal affective disorder, this might be a good option for you. And if your episodes of major depression are judged by you and your doctor to be relatively minor on depression scales, then possibly. But if you are suffering from anything more than mild depression or anxiety disorder, I would have to say no. In any case, since the herb only treats symptoms and not underlying cause, stressors, or coping skills, I would opt for a combination of St. John's Wort and psychotherapy—a combination that is certainly indicated in more severe mood disturbances.

I feel very strongly against giving my twelve-year-old drugs to treat his mild depression. I want to use St. John's Wort instead. What's an appropriate dose?

If you don't want to give your child "drugs," you should not be giving your child an herbal remedy. The fact that the FDA has not approved a botanical remedy as a drug doesn't mean it is safe to use. It can mean just the opposite in fact; that lack of definitive evidence about a substance's safety has so far prevented it from being stamped: Approved.

St. John's Wort has not been studied for its effects on children. You should have a powpow with a pediatrician familiar with your child's condition and overall health, and explore the many nondrug options available to you (see Chapter 3), before making the decision to include St. John's Wort in your child's treatment plan. If you, the doctor, and your child decide the risks are worthwhile, be sure you do not give young patients the full adult dose. If there's no effect, good or bad, after 6 weeks, you might increase the dose. But be aware it is your responsibility to monitor a child for side effects and weigh them against any benefits you may see your child obtaining. Do not under any circumstances put the burden of monitoring health on your child. Stay alert and be ready to discontinue use of St. John's Wort if any uncomfortable side effects appear.

If your doctor is unfamiliar with dosing of such herbal remedies for children, you might share this information obtained from various herbal references:

AGE	SUGGESTED DOSE
9–10	Half the adult dose
11–12	⅗ adult dose
13–14	⅘
15 and above	Full adult dose

Keep in mind your child's overall health, weight, and tolerance for other medications. Another dosing formula, called Clarke's rule, uses a ratio based on weight. It starts with the assumption of average adult weight as 150 pounds. The child's weight is then used to calculate his dose: if a child weighs fifty pounds ⅓ dose is indicated using this formula. In either case, such divided dosages are often easier to measure using liquid extracts (which can be administered mixed in a glass of orange juice), but look for those that use a glycerin rather than an alcohol base. To be blunt, however, I wouldn't treat my fifteen-year-old with St. John's Wort!

I'm borderline manic-depressive. I don't want to lose the highs, just deal with the lows. Can St. John's Wort do that?

You are definitely not alone in treasuring bipolar's "highs"—many of my patients struggle to find some combination of psychotherapy and mood stabilizers in combination with antidepressant to control the pits, but they complain of missing the manic creative heights of their disorder. Few people with this disorder have been clinically tested on St. John's Wort. These subjects did not note a recognizable improvement, although some anecdotal evidence exists that the herbal remedy helps soothe the disorder's lows during a depressive phase.

If it affects the depression, will St. John's Wort similarly "even out" the mania? I doubt it. Some sedative-like effects have been noted on milder forms of anxiety treated with the herb. Most researchers believe that bipolar disorder's two phases affect some of the same central nervous system centers, but that each phase also involves a separate set of biochemicals and functions.

I believe St. John's Wort might only work on your intentions to target the disorder's individual phases if you have a very distinct cycle of phases that is routinely separated by periods of health. This might give you time to bulk up on the herb's effects in time to combat depressive lows, but allow you time to taper off before a high is expected. Otherwise, the typical four-to-six-week period needed for the herb to begin its work may just work against you. Also, I would strongly recommend doing this under the supervision of your doctor and while taking a mood stabilizer.

And keep this note of caution in mind: Anxiety and nervous tension have been exhibited as side effects of therapy with St. John's Wort—not often, but the risk should be considered when bipolar or anxiety-disorder patients begin to debate the use of this herb in their treatment.

This sounds like some kind of miracle drug. Should I take it anyway, even if I'm not depressed? Will it make me feel even happier?

Aspirin is more of a "miracle drug" than St. John's Wort and even it is a long way from miraculous. No; it is never a good idea to dose with a remedy when you are not feeling the effects it is intended to treat. One reason is that St. John's Wort, like antidepressants, does not elevate mood in people not feeling depression's effects. If you are not emotionally or clinically depressed, then you will not get an extra emotional boost from dosing with St. John's Wort. Nothing will happen, except you might experience side effects. This leads to the second reason you should not use a therapy unless you have a condition: You are inviting side effects that have no accompanying benefit to outweigh them. If you weren't troubled by depression, why would you want to deal with upset stomach or dry mouth?

I'm not clinically depressed, I'm just feeling very sad over the recent death of my father. It's not bad enough for drugs, but I'd still like some help. Is St. John's Wort the answer?

If you were going through a "blue" period that you anticipated would lift in just a few weeks, I wouldn't recommend the herbal remedy since its effects would probably take too long to make an impact and might even introduce side effects just as you begin to feel emotionally well. The loss of a parent, however, especially one well loved or in situations where there were many unresolved issues, is a bereavement where you could expect to feel a mild state of the blues for some time—although not the disabling effects of true depression disorder. Talking about your feelings with loved ones or a counselor seems like a better idea in such a case. If your "very sad" feelings continue at the same pitch for more than a few weeks or begin to interfere with your day-to-day functioning, see a doctor. Together, you might determine that therapy with St. John's Wort was worth a try.

Is it true that St. John's Wort can be used to treat alcoholism?

Well, there is one small study that suggests there might be some relationship between St. John's Wort and alcohol-related depression. A study conducted by researchers in Ukraine suggests that St. John's Wort may treat the emotional toll of alcoholism as well as some of the disease's physical effects, such as chronic gastritis and peptic ulcers. However, those tempted to self-treat based on this cautious conclusion should be aware that the test involved only fifty-seven patients treated over a period of just two months. It would be very rash to assume any clear-cut relationship between St. John's Wort and a successful treatment of alcoholism until many more such studies are performed. In the meantime, the therapies that are successful begin by treating the addiction first and then the depression, which is typically lessened in any case once the primary disorder has been dealt with.

Bottom line, cards on the table—is this a good option for treating depression or not?

The bottom line, as I see it is this: I have *heard* about far more cases of depression helped by the drug than I have personally witnessed in my practice. I think one reason for this may be the simple fact that the people who come to see me or many other psychiatrists typically have more severe depression, or disorders complicated by some other factor, than do the majority of sufferers of depression. There is enough anecdotal evidence and clinical support for the herbal remedy's effectiveness, however, to make me cautiously optimistic for those with milder degrees of mood disorder.

I believe that one way to test out this herb's value is in combination with psychotherapy that addresses a person's coping mechanisms, strengthening them so that depression doesn't get quite as firm a grip. In that case, the biochemical malfunctions are being addressed as well as the impaired stress responses that so often weaken them. In addition, use of the herbal remedy to alleviate symptoms may release you from some of the more disabling effects enough to permit better application of the behavioral changes you need to make in psychotherapy. There's no doubt it is hard to concentrate and energize yourself to make behavioral changes when you are in pain.

Cards on the table, here are the roles I see for St. John's Wort in:

- **Dysthymia**—Yes, St. John's Wort might be a first line of treatment to try with this condition's more mild and chronic effects; how long the remedy might work is uncertain, however.
- **Mild episodes of depression disorder**—A qualified yes for St. John's Wort but only if symptoms are truly mild and the herbal remedy is taken under the guidance of a physician.
- **Moderate**—I am inclined to doubt St. John's Wort's efficacy in this range of mood disorder—or at least to count upon it. But the herb is a therapy to explore if conventional methods are not an option for some reason.
- **Severe depression**—*Do not attempt using St. John's Wort for these extreme disorders*; only one very limited documented study and little supporting anecdotal data exist that even suggest St. John's Wort has any effect on severe depression.
- **Seasonal affective disorder**—St. John's Wort looks like a viable option to augment light therapy or in cases where that therapy is not an option—again, only if symptoms are mild to moderate.
- **Bipolar disorder**—The herb may have some effect on bipolar's depressive lows, but its actions against mania symptoms are far less certain, and may actually enhance this phase; if your symptoms are severe for either phase, I would not recommend St. John's Wort at this time, and if the herb produces nervousness, discontinue use.
- **Sleep disorders**—A qualified yes for St. John's Wort use in the treatment of some of these disorders. If your problem is an inability to fall asleep in the first place or frequent awakenings, the herb will probably not help that insomnia; but for cases where sleep seems shallow and restless, St. John's Wort may be a an option for improving the relaxation levels and quality of your sleep.
- **Anxiety disorders**—Some studies suggest effectiveness against low-grade anxieties and symptoms of mild phobic

reaction; if you are obsessive-compulsive, schizophrenic, or suffer from post-traumatic stress disorder, there are far more certain and effective treatments you should explore—the herbal remedy may have no or a negative (nervousness-producing) effect.

These suggestions are simply guidelines to shape your approach to St. John's Wort. Discuss with your doctor how the cautions and information provided in this chapter coincide with your expression of mood disorder and overall treatment plan before you make any snap judgments about the use of St. John's Wort therapy.

SIX

❦

Beyond Depression:
Other Uses for St. John's Wort

If St. John's Wort could successfully treat even a fraction of the ailments it has been credited with, it would qualify as a miraculous medication. But before you get too excited, bear in mind that many of the herb's nondepression uses are only supported by anecdotal evidence, which means they have not been scientifically studied and documented, but simply passed along by word of mouth. People use a product, with varying levels of success, and they tell their friends, who then pass the tale on to others. Anecdotes like these can become like the child's game of "telephone," with odd interpretations and misinformation being passed on down the line. This can result in either alarmist reports inflating truly negligible risks (like the fears of phototoxicity attributed to St. John's Wort) or may grant miraculous properties to something that actually has little or no effect on a problem (like St. John's Wort's purported effects on weight loss). Even when anecdotal information is found to be true, such personal reports don't indicate how a medication will work on a broad spectrum of society, against variations of the same condition, or even on a second bout of the illness in the same person.

What you'll discover as you read through this chapter is that most of St. John's Wort's applications have no definitive body of evidence from clinical studies to support them. In some cases, the anecdotal evidence seems strong and has been passed down with convincing consistency through centuries. In other cases, its use is mentioned only by those who are selling the herb. So far, using St. John's Wort for any of these ailments appears safe, when conducted under the care of a physician familiar with you and your condition, and when the herb is taken in normal doses. Thus, a short ''trial'' of St. John's Wort is likely to fall within Hippocrates' oath to first ''do no harm.''

Sometimes, though, placing unwarranted trust in an herb can prevent you from seeking other treatment, for which there may be documented proof of effectiveness. Your condition could get worse in that case, or not improve as quickly or as dramatically under another kind of therapy.

Taking St. John's Wort can also generate a false sense of well-being—a ''feeling'' that you're going to get better that could trick you into engaging in activities that are actually inappropriate or harmful for you. Finally, and most importantly, *see your physician* before making a self-diagnosis about any of these conditions. Sometimes a condition that seems relatively mild—like a rash, belly pains, or periodic dizzy spells—can mask a more serious disorder that requires immediate attention. When it comes to your self-treatment do not assume you know what you're dealing with until other causes for your symptoms have been ruled out.

That's just one of the many reasons I always caution people to apply alternative therapies under the guidance of a physician. However, I also warn them that there are so many new treatments physicians need to stay updated on that your doctor may not have all the current facts about St. John's Wort or another therapy you might be interested in. That leaves a large burden of your own care on you.

Be vigilant when on any kind of therapy—conventional or alternative. Keep a record of your reactions while on the treatment. This includes both physical changes and emotional ones. Ask family and friends to let you know if they notice any changes as well. Use your judgment—and trust your instincts. If something ''just doesn't feel right,'' let your doctor know immediately. More often than not, patients catch on to early-warning signs of problems before their doctors spot them. You live with your body every day and will know better than anyone else when it's not working properly. Your doctor can help you to determine if this is a normal reaction to the drug or not.

When it comes to alternative treatments like St. John's Wort, vigilance is even more important. Because individual reactions to the herb may not be well documented for the many and varied uses addressed in this chapter, you'll have to watch carefully to see how your body chemistry interacts with the herb for any of these ailments. Judge whether the healing effects are worth the price you are paying for the herb and the associated effects with regular use. Give any therapy a fair shot (in the case of St. John's Wort effects might not show up for two to six weeks), but don't beat a dead horse in your search for a natural solution. If St. John's Wort is not working, it is appropriate and wise to seek other medical options, some of which are suggested here. Remember that some commercial drug preparations, such as antibiotics, morphine, digitalis, quinine, reserpine, and some anticarcinogens, are themselves derived from plant sources and merely concentrate the active ingredients of natural remedies.

(Before using St. John's Wort for any of the purposes noted in this chapter, carefully read the cautions about possible interactions with food and other medications in Chapter Four—Is St. John's Wort Safe and Effective? Use the information about St. John's Wort in Chapter Seven to help you choose the correct preparation for your specific needs.)

And, since many people seek alternative treatments for their children, work with your child's pediatrician to determine the correct dose of St. John's Wort. *Never* give a child the same amount of medication you would give an adult without consulting a physician, no matter how innocent-seeming or "natural" the source may seem. Herbal remedies can be strong medicines, they can be toxic in excessive doses, and they should be treated with the same care you would give any drug in the hands of children. The same caution should be used when applying St. John's Wort remedies to older people and to women who are pregnant or nursing.

I've heard this thing can cure everything from worms to heart disease to the common cold. But is there *any* scientific proof of its effects on illnesses beside depression?

Some of the nondepression treatments attributed to St. John's Wort have actually been the subject of testing, both in the United States and abroad, especially in Germany, the countries of the former Soviet Union and France. However, many of the European tests were not conducted to the standards of our own Food and Drug Administration (FDA), which ensures that strict controls and guidelines are employed in clinical studies to ensure that a medication is safe and effective—even if long-term side effects do sometimes provide an unpleasant surprise later. The tests on St. John's Wort have most notably focused upon its effects on wounds, mutated cells (like those found in cancers), cardiac functions (like the passage of electrical impulses that control the rhythm and beating of the heart), and various viruses (everything from the common cold to Epstein-Barr, herpes simplex, and AIDS/HIV). Unless specifically noted, however, assume that the applications for St. John's Wort described in this chapter are based only on anecdotal evidence.

A short biology refresher course: The nervous system is the conglomerate formed by your brain, spinal cord, and all the peripheral nerves in your body. Nerves form a complex network of vinelike branches that extend from your scalp to the tips of your fingers and toes. They are the highways for "impulses," messages carrying information about sensory input to your spinal cord and brain, as well as the reflexive and willful responses to these sensations. These could consist of messages about temperature, pain, light, sound, taste, smell, or the need for small motor movements. The movements it controls are both voluntary, like scratching an itch on your leg, or involuntary, the classic patellar tendon reflex (knee jerk). In a healthy system, nerve impulses travel at speeds of up to 350 feet per second.

Is St. John's Wort a nervine? And do nervines act like tranquilizers?

The term nervine is used in herbal jargon to refer to a plant-based therapy that soothes disorders related to the nervous system. The role played by nervines is as multilayered as the complex nervous system itself.

Because the nervous system is so broad in its effects, nervines are almost too broad a category. To make plant-action identification less confusing, the nervines are generally divided into three subcategories: tonics, relaxants, and stimulants. These three can be divided even more by their actions on the various body systems: circulatory (blood flow), respiratory (breathing), urinary (passage of liquid waste), reproductive (sexual organs), digestive (processing of fuels), or musculoskeletal (muscles, skin, and skeleton). St. John's Wort is classified as both a tonic and relaxant. The two actions have similar but slightly different effects.

From an herbalist's perspective, tonics offer support to a nervous system under strain, strengthening it or "feeding" it in a variety of ways intended to help revitalize the entire system. They essentially perform a damage-control function. In theory, nervous tissues harmed by stress, traumatic shock, or a neurological or psychiatric condition can be repaired though the use of nervine tonics. Tonics are considered a long-term therapy, to help boost the very basics of the nervous system.

Nervine relaxants produce more sedative-like effects. St. John's Wort is often credited with a tranquilizing action that aids the battered nervous system during times of crisis, like periods of increased stress, anxiety, grief or confusion—any situation that "ties" your emotions into "knots." Relaxants should only be used as a short-term therapy, though, to soothe you over a hump by temporarily reducing responses to stress and strain. The danger here is to overuse the tranquilizing effect of these relaxants. Most people believe that it's far better to address the underlying emotions and situations causing the stress than simply to relieve the symptoms produced by those feelings and environments. However, sometimes the former can only begin after the relaxant has taken the edge off the stress—allowing you the luxury of addressing the concerns rather than giving in to the emotional swell.

Many nervines have other qualities as well—some may have pain-relieving properties, perform as hypnotics or act as antispasmodics, although the latter quality is probably more likely to result from direct effects on smooth muscles rather than nerve tissue. You should therefore choose your herbal therapy by looking at your various symptoms and choosing the single herb which addresses most or all of them. If the rumors indeed prove true, and St. John's Wort is eventually revealed to have real effects on the many ailments that have been claimed *and* on depression, it could have a twofold effect on depression. If your depression stemmed from the suffering of chronic sciatic pain or a viral infection, for instance, the herb might treat both conditions. An exciting thought—but still just an idea, not a fact.

I was in an accident that damaged my pelvic nerves. Can St. John's Wort help?

Damage to nerves is an all-too-common result of pelvic injury, usually because a nerve bundle has been lacerated or crushed. Recovery usually occurs in all but the most severe cases, but may take anywhere from three months to two years. In the meantime, people often look for other resources to help deal with the pain. St. John's Wort has had a long history in the treatment of virtually all disorders involving the nervous system, and I have seen numerous anecdotal references to its effectiveness on problems in the pelvic area. If the herb is effective for a post-traumatic nerve disorder, it may be because of its anti-inflammatory and analgesic actions, which have been noted in some Russian studies, but are mostly supported by strong word-of-mouth accounts. I have also seen St. John's Wort recommended for other pelvic problems that are presumed to result from nervous tension. Although pelvic pain is sometimes associated with depression or anxiety, I would not have great confidence in this application.

Before self-treating for pelvic problems, sufferers should be examined by a physician to rule out other causes for the pain, such as pelvic inflammatory disease (also known as PID or salpingitis), a sexually transmitted disease, irritable bowel syndrome, endometriosis, or urethritis, among others. Some of these conditions, while not originating in the pelvic region, may cause pain to present in that area and should be treated with other therapies, including antibiotic drugs, relaxation exercises, biofeedback, and hormonal therapies, or surgery. Prompt treatment with the proper medication is sometimes essential in preventing risk of permanent effects such as sterility, which can result from PID—so be sure your condition is properly diagnosed. In some cases, pelvic pain is a result of physical or emotional trauma from current or past sexual abuse, a situation which should certainly be addressed by more comprehensive methods than herbal remedies.

What is an anti-inflammatory? I feel I should already know what it means.

That's probably because it's one of those terms that gets thrown around a lot without anyone really being aware of what it means. Anti-inflammatories reduce—you guessed it—inflammation, which is just the term describing the way your body's tissues respond to injury or invasion (e.g., arthritis, pancreatitis, hepatitis, or dermatitis). This often "angry" or flamelike reaction can produce swelling, sensations of heat, redness, and varying levels of pain. In extreme cases, inflammation can cause a loss of the affected organ's functions. The level of your body's reaction can fluctuate radically, based on the agent causing the inflammation, your relative health, and the area of the body affected. It can also be temporary or chronic, occurring with debilitating frequency and severity.

Rheumatoid and degenerative arthritis are well-known types of inflammation of the joints, but literally every type of tissue or organ system can be affected. Aspirin and ibuprofen are among the more common anti-inflammatories. In herbalism, herbs are not considered true anti-inflammatories, since the intent is not to stop the body from reacting in an appropriate way to invasion or injury, but to help soothe the uncomfortable effects of the inflammation and to help target the root cause of your body's reaction. When taken as anti-inflammatories for conditions other than dermatitis, herbs are generally applied internally, using alcohol- or glycerin-based tinctures.

St. John's Wort is an antispasmodic? What does an antispasmodic do?

St. John's Wort has been said to be antispasmodic in anecdotal accounts and in herbal therapies, although this use has not been clinically proven. The cramping and spasms produced by tightened, clenched muscles can be eased and sometimes even prevented by herbals of this type. Antispasmodics are classed by their actions on specific systems, like the muscles controlling the circulatory, reproductive, digestive, or nervous system.

Herbs with this action help calm the peripheral nerves sending impulses to the brain, as well as relax muscle tissue. The herb's alleged effects on digestive problems and menstrual cramping could be due to this antispasmodic action. When antispasmodic effects are combined with the herb's nervine, or sedative, qualities, you may have the ingredients for an overall relaxant. Before you give up your regular sessions with the physical therapist, though, see if these effects appear with your own use of the herb, as they have not been proven. In addition, be aware that many medications only perform their therapeutic functions when a problem exists in the first place— in other words, if your pain is not from inflammation, you probably won't feel any of the beneficial effects.

I know headache remedies are analgesics, but St. John's Wort is also. Does that mean it's a headache treatment?

An analgesic is a medication that deadens *any* kind of pain, not just headaches. St. John's Wort is considered an analgesic herb because of its effects on many types of pain. Moreover, some believe that St. John's Wort can work as a therapy for tension headaches. Of course, this could be due as much to the herb's effects on the depression and anxieties that are so often associated with tension headaches. The herb is not used in the treatment of vascular headaches such as migraine, which in theory might even be aggravated by St. John's Wort. In fact, the herb may slow metabolism of the amino acid tyramine, which can frequently trigger a migraine headache, so is therefore not indicated for that condition. If you want to treat migraine or headache with an herbal remedy, a better choice might be applications of the plant feverfew. And there are now many prescription drugs that are quite effective for migraine, such as Imitrex, Propanolol, and Divalproex.

What other types of pains can St. John's Wort treat as an analgesic?

There is some evidence that St. John's Wort works as a topical analgesic for wounds and arthritic joints. More anecdotal evidence suggests St. John's Wort can be taken to lessen the pain of a toothache, sciatica, or hemorrhoids as well—

virtually any pain associated with nerves has been mentioned at one time or another in relation to this herb. Some believe that the chemical hyperforin, found in St. John's Wort, is largely responsible for these painkilling effects. I prefer to take aspirin, ibuprofen, or acetominophen, however, because they are much better studied, more readily available, and, in generic form, less expensive than St. John's Wort. To each her own!

I'm desperate to find something for my menstrual cramps. Is St. John's Wort the answer?

Because of its supposed analgesic, antispasmodic and anti-inflammatory effects, St. John's Wort could turn out to be a viable alternative treatment for painful menstrual cramps. It relaxes tissues in the reproductive system and may reduce swelling. This use, too, comes to us mainly through anecdotal information, but does date back to very old sources. There are other ways St. John's Wort could help women with their menstrual cycles, too. St. John's Wort has been noted for its diuretic actions, reducing the water-weight gain that can be uncomfortable and even painful for some women. As an antidepressant, St. John's Wort may also prevent or treat the depression and emotional fluctuations that many women contend with each month. Finally, it appears that St. John's Wort may help reduce levels of estrogen, which may also help explain the herb's apparent actions on menstrual and menopausal troubles.

I'm going through menopause with all its attendant joys. I'm taking St. John's Wort and heard it has an effect on varicose veins as well as menopausal blues. Dare I hope?

Buried among St. John's Wort's constituents are chemicals called phytosterols. These feature a nucleus that is steroidlike in structure. How these "agri-steroids" may affect humans once they are ingested is still unknown, but some scientists think there might be some connection to hormonal conditions and disorders, and would classify medications or herbs with this effect as "estrogenic" or "hormonal" therapies. As has been noted, St. John's Wort may impact on estrogen levels in some way. That might account for the herb's recommendation as a treatment for women experiencing menopause. Or its antidepressant effects may be the sole action of St. John's Wort in the treatment of menopausal symptoms.

Studies have shown that in Western society, where age, especially among women, does not garner the respect and authority it earns in many other cultures, women going through menopause may be more likely to experience self-doubts, a sense of being "over the hill," or moodiness. St. John's Wort could help with these feelings during the period of menopause, and is listed in the British Pharmacopoeia as a therapy for "menopausal neuroses." Although this name sounds alarming, we don't have any conditions with this name. Other herbs that crop up as therapies to manage symptoms of menopause include black cohosh (a diuretic and treatment for hot flashes produced when hormones are released periodically into the blood), *Vitex* (more commonly called chaste tree or chaste berry, for hot flashes, vaginal dryness, and depression), and Dong Quai (a Chinese herb used as a tonic and antispasmodic).

As for the use of St. John's Wort in the treatment of varicose veins, here again we enter the realm of purely anecdotal evidence. St. John's Wort *is* listed in herbal literature as a therapy for this condition, which is the result of enlarged or distorted veins popping up "superficially" from just under the skin. Varicose veins are most often found in the lower extremities, although they can also be present internally, as hemorrhoids. Varicose veins are caused by poor functioning of certain valves. Women are particularly susceptible to this condition because of the added risks of pregnancy and sitting with crossed legs, which puts added pressure on these veins. Instead of using dubious herbal remedies for this condition, you might consider involving more exercise in your routine, avoiding the crossed-leg posture, breaking up long sessions of sitting by moving around, and eating foods that do not clog your cardiovascular system, like those low in saturated fats and carbohydrates.

When taken for menopausal depression or hormonal effects, St. John's Wort is usually administered in the form of a tincture or tea. For the topical treatment of varicose veins, however, it needs to be applied externally, through an oil, cream, or balm.

I know "emmenagogue" has something to do with the menstrual cycle, but what? Is St. John's Wort an emmenagogue?

St. John's Wort is sometimes described as an emmenagogue. Generally, this term is applied to herbs that promote a more regular menstrual flow, but there is no scientific evidence to support such an action by St. John's Wort. However, if the word is used to describe a remedy that soothes the reproductive system as a whole, St. John's Wort could be classified as an emmenagogue because of the effects previously described.

Is it true that St. John's Wort can soothe acute pains like sciatica?

Sciatica is a form of neuralgia, a pain traveling along the length of a nerve. Neuralgia can originate from a variety of sources that spark inflammation. These can range from a poor diet (rare in 1998) or lack of exercise to infection or bone-related problems. Sometimes it begins with the onset of a disease, like tuberculosis, malaria, or tetanus.

Neuralgia, or neuritis, can take many forms. Anyone afflicted with sciatica knows just how debilitating this particular type of chronic pain can be. Compression of the sciatic nerve, such as that produced by a ruptured disk, can send pain streaking down through the hips, along the back of the thigh and around the foot. Even prolonged sitting on an overstuffed wallet can set off a bout of sciatica. The pain can sometimes be felt in areas of the body untouched by the nerve itself, a sensation called referred pain, which can confuse patients as to exactly what kind of condition they are experiencing. See a doctor if you suffer this kind of chronic pain—if it is the result of a ruptured disk, surgery may be required.

Rest, applied heat, and other physical therapy may soothe the irritated nerve in acute cases, as can gently stretching the leg or using corrective shoes. If you are taking St. John's Wort as a remedy for sciatica, it is usually applied externally, as an oil or other liniment. However, some herbal sources also recommend drinking St. John's Wort tea. Use of the herb for neuralgia is so far anecdotal, so there is no definitive source to settle the question of which application is best.

My arthritis is mild, but painful all the same. Can St. John's Wort give me relief?

Arthritis is caused by inflammation in a joint and is considered a disease of the musculoskeletal system. The inflammation causes friction between the bones that meet at the joint. That sounds painful and it is; moreover, the condition often becomes chronic. The broad term of rheumatism applies to inflammations of not only joints, but muscles and tendons as well. More specific classifications of these conditions occur, too, such as gout.

Gout is a form of acute arthritis brought about by crystal-like deposits on a joint and excess levels of uric acid in the blood; it results from an inherited abnormality in uric-acid metabolism. Despite common wisdom, gout is not caused by overly rich diets or obesity. St. John's Wort pops up in herbal lists for the treatment of both the more general and specific of these rheumatic conditions. The herb's anti-inflammatory and analgesic properties both apply; and alkaloids in the herb have also been credited with antirheumatic effects. The recommended application is massaging St. John's Wort oil onto the afflicted areas, but regular dosing with tea made from the herb has been promoted as well. However, you should consult a physician about taking other, more potent analgesics, exercise within your limitations, and watch your diet. Arthritic inflammation is spurred by the buildup of toxins in the system, so consume more fruits and green or root vegetables, and avoid red meats if you suffer from this.

I've seen St. John's Wort described as an aromatic herb. Does that just mean it smells good?

Actually, yes, that's one meaning of the word—but be warned, aromatics may simply have a powerful odor, not necessarily an attractive one. Fortunately, the aroma given off by the St. John's Wort is not unpleasant. Medicinally, as is rumored in the case of St. John's Wort, it may also indicate an herb that stimulates the digestive process.

I suffer from "nervous stomach" but St. John's Wort seems to help. Is it all in my mind?

St. John's Wort's soothing effects have been noted anecdotally for a variety of conditions related to the digestive system. These include ulcers, gastritis, diarrhea, and nausea, as well as "nervous stomach," a condition that may actually relate to the colon. Again, the antispasmodic actions of St. John's Wort may take the credit here. By relaxing cramped muscles involved in the functions of the stomach and intestinal tract St. John's Wort can promote the smoother passage of food and wastes. "Carminative" effects are those which calm the ache of stomach pain and reduce gas in the digestive system. St. John's Wort may work in this way, thanks to its combination of volatile oils. The herb's soothing actions may be in your mind to a certain extent, though—in the sense that St. John's Wort can alleviate the stress which so often prompts intestinal troubles. Of course, a placebo effect is not out of the question here, either, since these effects are all largely anecdotal.

I have dysentery. Is St. John's Wort the healthy way to go?

Well, it's one way to go. St. John's Wort has been recommended in herbal texts as a therapy for the assortment of intestinal disorders collectively called dysentery. These conditions most often target the colon—also known as the large intestine—and are caused by inflamed mucous membranes. Dysentery may be caused by worms (more about this follows), infections brought about by exposure to bacteria or viruses, or by chemical contaminants. Like the other intestinal disorders, diet plays an important role in dysentery. In addition to any herbal remedies you might try for these conditions, a change in diet is indicated—steer clear of foods that haven't been stored correctly (fruits about to spoil, badly refrigerated leftovers, or stuff left in cabinets too long), drinking too much liquid with meals (especially liquor, caffeinated beverages, and water that hasn't been properly filtered) or living in unsanitary conditions. A lighter diet and bed rest will help, as will reducing intake of laxatives. If taking St. John's Wort for intestinal troubles, try the teas first before using other forms of the herb.

Can St. John's Wort really work as a diuretic?

That can't be answered as definitively as you might like since studies have not been focused on this particular use of the herb. However, patients have informally traded information on St. John's Wort actions as a diuretic. Diuretics are often used by women during menstrual cycles to reduce the amount of water weight gained at that time. They promote this type of weight loss because diuretics speed the process by which water, sodium, and other trace chemicals are eliminated from the body. In addition to the discomfort caused by fluid retention, more serious problems can arise from excessive fluids stored in the tissues, a condition known as edema. For these more serious conditions affecting the heart, liver, and kidney, you should receive a doctor's care, and you should not try St. John's Wort unless conventional therapies have been exhausted. But to alleviate simple water retention caused by nonthreatening conditions, by all means try a tea or other internal application of St. John's Wort.

I've heard St. John's Wort causes nausea and that it cures it. Which is true?

There are a few scattered, anecdotal accounts of people successfully using St. John's Wort as an antiemetic, a medication that prevents vomiting or helps alleviate feelings of nausea. However, there are more reports of gastrointestinal upset, sometimes associated with feelings of nausea, which are described by people taking the herb. Sensations of nausea were most often reported by patients using St. John's Wort at the same time as potent MAOI (monoamine oxidase inhibitor) medications or those using large amounts of the herb. This is probably related to the herb's effects on serotonin in the gut or brainstem, since similar side effects are reported by people taking certain antidepressants. Nausea is not a common side effect, however, for people using the herb in proper doses.

I've heard St. John's Wort described as an expectorant. What effect does that action have on coughs, colds, and a runny nose?

There are some anecdotal claims that St. John's Wort acts as an expectorant. Typically, this term refers to medications that help rid the lungs and throat of mucus that clogs them when you have a cold or other upper-respiratory infection. I've run across numerous anecdotal accounts of St. John's Wort's effectiveness for coughs and colds, which indicate it could work as an expectorant, but it's also possible that the herb acts less as a thinner of mucus than as a "relaxing expectorant," a subcategory with an action similar to antispasmodics, with the therapeutic effect of calming the bronchial spasms that produce coughs. The herb's anti-inflammatory actions could also play a role in colds, reducing swelling of nose, throat, and lung tissues. Finally, St. John's Wort has "demulcent" qualities. This term describes oil-like therapies that act as balms to soothe sore skin. The herb's volatile oils can have demulcent effects on irritated throats and raw noses.

Treatment with herbal remedies is pretty common for coughs and colds—people routinely use teas labeled as balms for sore throats, or cold care. Zinc, a common metallic element, is gaining some attention in this area, too. And *Echinacea* is another herb besides St. John's Wort that is a commonly accepted herbal remedy. These therapies probably can't hurt, and enough people have traded stories of relief to suggest they could help. But don't rely on them if your cold is severe, or if symptoms seem to move from high in your chest and throat to deeper in your lungs. Congestion from a simple cold can lead to a more serious infection, such as sinusitis, bronchitis, or pneumonia. So see a doctor as soon as possible if symptoms persist beyond a week, if you feel lousier than you normally do with a cold, you have trouble breathing, you feel pain in your chest, you have a fever, the lymph glands in your neck or under your jaw feel swollen, you begin vomiting or get chills, urine is dark, or if your throat, skin, or eyes appear yellow. Ear infections and strep throat also could hit a person whose immune system is weakened by a cold, so be alert to any changes in your condition. In children, frequent bouts with colds could indicate the presence of allergies, so get your child checked if this is a persistent condition.

So St. John's Wort may work on colds. But can it help something as serious as heart disease?

Just how great an impact is uncertain, but it appears that herbs like St. John's Wort could have beneficial effects on your cardiovascular system. It is known that bioflavonoids like quercetin and rutin act on tiny blood vessels, helping to improve the strength of capillary walls to reduce the potential for leaks, called hemorrhages. The strength of capillaries is vitally important to the cardiovascular system, even though they are so tiny, since it is at this level that oxygen and wastes are exchanged between blood and tissues. One study, reported in the *British Medical Journal*, classified the herb as a vasoactive medication, which means it can affect the diameter of blood vessels. It received this label as a result of effects on coronary arteries measured in the test. Procyanidin was the constituent being isolated and observed in that test, but some of the herb's other constituents may also affect the cardiovascular system. Another recent test reported some effects on cardiac conduction, the system of nerve signals that regulates the pumping rhythms of your heart. This effect needs to be confirmed in further studies but holds promise that rumors of St. John's Wort's effects on the heart are not as far-fetched as they may sound. Before attempting to self-treat a condition as serious as heart disease, however, seek the advice of your physician or a heart specialist—the sooner, the better. Some herbs have powerful cardiac effects, and it should be recalled that digitalis originally was extracted from the foxglove plant, so be very careful using any remedies not prescribed by your doctor. Since so few studies have been made in this area using St. John's Wort, extreme caution is indicated.

If St. John's Wort helps strengthen blood vessels, can it help with anemia?

St. John's Wort may have some effect on the condition known as anemia, but not so much from its capillary-strengthening actions as by its stimulation of hemoglobin production. Hemoglobin is the molecule that carries oxygen within the red blood cells. It appears that one of the herb's constituents can help your body make more of this important protein-iron compound. Anemia is a condition in which the number of red blood cells or the amount of hemoglobin is too low to supply the oxygen your body requires. But before beginning treatment of anemia with St. John's Wort or another therapy, see a doctor. Since anemia is itself merely a description of some more specific disorder, you need a doctor to determine the condition's root cause. For example, is the anemia caused by an illness that reduces the production of new blood cells, speeds the destruction of red blood cells, causes the loss of too many blood cells, a deficiency of dietary iron, or one of the several vitamins necessary to make red blood cells? More effective treatments than St. John's Wort that target the true source of the anemia could include drugs to stimulate production of marrow, antibiotics, vitamin treatments, iron supplements, dosing with ascorbic acid or, in more extreme cases, transfusions. Of course, an anemia caused by blood loss ultimately will require identifying and, if possible, fixing the source of the bleeding.

I've heard that St. John's Wort can purify blood transfusions. Can that possibly be true?

There was a recent report in the journal *Transfusions* that holds promise that one of the herb's constituents, hypericin, could have a cleansing action on blood transfusions. The hypericin used in this study had been enhanced by exposure to light. The study reflected interest in hypericin's antiviral effects and showed that by preventing viruses from binding to and entering healthy cells, hypericin could end the spread of infection. Exciting, yes. Definitive, no. *Much* more testing needs to be done to determine the viability of this use of the herb's ingredient.

My son is a chronic bed wetter. Can St. John's Wort help? I don't want to try something as serious as drug therapy.

Before you use St. John's Wort or other therapies to address this problem—called nocturnal enuresis—first be sure a problem really exists. Most physicians will not treat enuresis until a child is at least six years old, as it is still considered age-appropriate to wet overnight until that age. But if your child is over six years old and has rarely had a dry night (this is called primary enuresis) or if your child had been dry for at least three to six months but has suddenly begun wetting again (called secondary enuresis), then consult a pediatrician. Your child's doctor can rule out organic diseases for which enuresis is a symptom, like diabetes or a bladder problem. Once it has been established that no such primary disorder exists, you can work together with your child, the doctor, and your family to develop a plan to help your child stay dry. St. John's Wort has been mentioned in the herbal literature and occasionally in anecdotal reports as a treatment—both as a tea drunk in small amounts at night and as an oil rubbed into the inner thighs—but this use has not been scientifically demonstrated. Perhaps the herb's nervous-system actions stimulate the nerves in the bladder to send their messages that the bladder is full. Or it may turn out that St. John's Wort has some effect on the production of a hormone known as antidiuretic hormone (ADH), which kicks in at night to concentrate the volume of urine by cutting down on water content.

Recent studies have shown that some children who experience enuresis do not produce this hormone at night. But before placing faith in a remedy surrounded by so many question marks, try some of the therapies recommended by the National Enuresis Society to address the various suspected causes of the problem: To enlarge the capacity of a bladder that may be smaller than normal, children are advised to hold their urine as long as possible during the day to gradually stretch the bladder. To stimulate the wake-up call of a full bladder in children who sleep too soundly, moisture alarms in the underpants or bed linens are used to sound when a child begins to wet. Sometimes simply including your child in the changing of bed linens and washing of wet clothes helps, too, as long as it is not treated as a punishment. Involving your child in the consequences of enuresis can help motivate dedication to other therapies and will help lighten the load on other family members—something that will also reassure the young bed wetter.

Your concern about drug therapy is understandable. Some doctors prescribe tricyclic antidepressants for the treatment of enuresis—their actions on bed wetting may result from delaying the initiation of starting urination (which also may cause urinary retention when tricyclics are used with adults for treatment of other conditions) and, perhaps, lightening the child's level of sleep across the night. But other side effects of tricyclic therapy in children are less beneficial and potentially dangerous, so their use is limited—especially since relapses after a child comes off the drug are almost certain. Use caution and monitor your child carefully when on these powerful drugs. A hormone supplement, known as Desmopressin or DDAVP, is a synthetic form of antidiuretic hormone. Its side effects (few have been noted) are far less of a risk than those of tricyclics, but like the drugs, the hormone is only a temporary solution—as many as 90% of children go back to wetting after stopping the medication. Some families use the hormone to help ensure children stay dry while at sleepaway camp or on overnight visits.

Your pediatrician may have other ideas for using positive reinforcement in the treatment of enuresis, and that's the way to go. Don't use threats, punishment, or ridicule against a child who wets—evidence shows it will not speed a "cure" and that it may produce emotional or behavioral problems in addition to the enuresis, which is not a psychological disorder. Children do not intend to wet the bed out of spite, anger, or stress, so scolding them has no effect. And be sure your child knows he or she is not alone: Between five and seven million children share this problem, according to the NES. If you choose to use St. John's Wort to help combat enuresis, talk to your doctor about appropriate doses—children should never be given the same amounts of herbal remedies as an adult. Since the tea is usually administered right before bedtime for this condition, be aware St. John's Wort might exacerbate the problem if it doesn't fix it.

I am an adult and ashamed to admit I have trouble controlling my bladder. It seems crazy, but I heard St. John's Wort can help.

It's a sad fact that adults who suffer from urinary incontinence are often embarrassed to admit to it; sometimes they won't even inform a doctor of the problem. But many men and women suffer from this condition, either after surgery such as radical prostatectomy or as a result of pregnancy, childbirth, trauma to the head or spinal cord, and diseases involving the kidney. Sometimes the problem is temporary, but even so there are treatments that may help, particularly a series of exercises designed to strengthen the muscles surrounding the bladder, urethra, vagina, and sphincter, a muscle system called the pelvic floor muscles. These strengthening movements are called Kegel exercises and when performed correctly can make a significant difference in bladder control for incontinent men and women. There are other treatments you and your doctor may consider, including bladder training, hormone supplements, and some alpha-adrenergic agonists, anticholinergic, or antidepressant drugs. Perhaps because it may share the effects of some of these commercial medications, St. John's Wort is sometimes used by people to treat urinary incontinence. I've run across a few anecdotal reports of St. John's Wort as a successful remedy, but that and some herbal references are the only evidence I've seen so far in support of this use.

What are worms? Is it what it sounds like? Can St. John's Wort help?

Yes, worms are just what they sound like—parasitic tapeworms (different varieties are found in fish, pork, and beef), threadworms, hookworms, pinworms or roundworms (not to be confused with the skin condition known as ringworm). These parasites find their way into a person's skin or intestinal tract through exposure to soil contaminated with human waste or by eating meats that have not been thoroughly cooked. It's every bit as unpleasant as it sounds, but is not usually life-threatening. Dosing with St. John's Wort tea or its other internal applications has been noted in herbal references for this condition. But if you or your child has been diagnosed with worms, there are other remedies that have better documented success, including the use of prescription treatments like Vermox, Mebendazole, Piperazine, and Pyrantel pamoate.

Children are most often the victims of infestation, because they walk barefoot a lot more and generally have less concern about hygiene than adults. Children should be treated by a physician for this condition—do not medicate with St. John's Wort until you have talked with your pediatrician about appropriate therapies. Some precautions to discuss: some worms can leave the body in the warmth of a bed, so check the sheets after your child has gone to sleep and, of course, kill any that emerge. Rigorous cleaning of the environment of the infected person is also necessary—wash any sheets, towels, clothes, or other fabrics that come in contact with him or her, likewise scrub toilets and tubs, encourage meticulous hand-washing, and keep family members apart if one is infected during the period of treatment (or you might want to preventively dose the whole household).

Tell me St. John's Wort works on jaundice.

I wish I could be so definitive, but I can't. This condition is caused by inflammation of the liver and is characterized by yellowing of the eyes, mucous membranes, and skin from excessive amounts of bilirubin, an orangish yellow pigment found in bile. Hepatitis is most commonly caused by viral infections and can develop into chronic and life-threatening forms. Jaundice can also be caused by obstruction of the bile ducts by gallstones or a tumor. Apart from a series of mentions in herbals, and some historical references to this action, no evidence exists to support this claim. The effects St. John's Wort may have on jaundice have not been clinically studied or even officially documented. Thus, St. John's Wort should never be used to treat jaundice unless all credible medical avenues have been explored.

Does St. John's Wort act as a hepatic? I've heard it works on liver conditions.

"Hepatic" is the traditional term given to herbs that "strengthen" the functions of the liver. As discussed above, the liver produces bile, which ancient physicians considered an essential ingredient in determining health and emotional well-being. In truth, as the largest organ in the body (excluding the skin), the liver's actions affect so many functions that its smooth operation does have a tremendous impact on your overall well-being. In addition to the production of bile (which prepares fats for digestion), the liver also helps to process hemoglobin, vitamins, glucose, and proteins. Perhaps most importantly, the liver breaks down or metabolizes potentially toxic substances, including alcohol and nicotine, and poisonous chemicals produced in the body itself. No studies exist on St. John's Wort's effects as a hepatic. Frankly, I don't think this old-fashioned term has any relevance to modern medicine. St. John's Wort may have gained this reputation because of alleged effects on jaundice, a condition brought about by diseases of the liver.

There was some improvement reported in the symptoms of hepatitis experienced by some HIV-infected patients in San Francisco being tested for the antiviral effects of St. John's Wort. These reports were not central to the study's findings, however, and are hardly definitive. And, in fact, patients with liver problems might need to exercise caution when using the herb, since a few anecdotal accounts of liver-related problems have cropped up in regard to St. John's Wort. No clinical studies have noted this side effect to any degree of certainty, but it may be something to watch for. Any strong medication, which could be construed as a harmful substance by your body, could impact on the liver's toxin-cleansing functions.

I'm a runner and I use St. John's Wort to treat my minor sprains and bruises. Am I the only one who's discovered this?

Sorry, but you are far from the first to recognize the herb's effectiveness as a treatment for bruises. St. John's Wort is often listed in herbals as a therapy for the speedy healing of bruises, also known as contusions, as well as black eyes. Bruises are injuries that don't break the skin or produce an external wound, but instead damage the soft tissues, and are characterized by swelling, tenderness or pain, and discoloration on the skin. St. John's Wort's anti-inflammatory actions may take care of the swelling when it is gently rubbed onto the bruise in a cream or oil. The herb's effects on capillaries could speed repair of damaged blood vessels under the skin—it is the decomposing blood from this hemorrhaging that produces the colorful effect of a bruise. In addition to treatment with St. John's Wort, cold compresses can help reduce swelling if applied immediately after the blow. *Arnica* is another herbal remedy popularly prescribed for bruising or sprains. But *Arnica* is not to be used on bruises where the skin is also broken, and many herbalists recommend St. John's Wort as a better herbal choice for damage to those body parts crammed with nerves, like the hands, feet, and back.

I've heard that St. John's Wort may act as an antibiotic. This may sound dumb, but what exactly does an antibiotic do?

When it comes to things medical there's no such entity as a dumb question. We use terms like antibiotic every day without really knowing what they mean. An antibiotic kills bacteria, plain and simple. A bacteriostatic stops the growth of microorganisms that could cause illness. These microorganisms commonly enter the body through the air via cuts or other breaks in the skin.

Why is St. John's Wort called an astringent?

St. John's Wort has high levels of tannins, which help in the herb's astringent action. Basically, astringents promote the separation of proteins, which causes tissues under the skin to contract, or pucker. That action could help prevent loss of blood and other fluids from wounds or other breaks in the skin. It also produces a numbing effect which can help alleviate pain. Astringents are also present in the digestive system. There, the clenching effects may reduce inflammation, which in turn may help reduce diarrhea.

Can you use St. John's Wort creams as emollients?

Yes, St. John's Wort can help soothe skin broken by rashes, inflammation, or minor burns, which is what an emollient does. Some emollients also promote softening of the skin. St. John's Wort's potential value as a cosmetic skin softener has not been addressed or widely noted anecdotally. But it is useful when spread over cuts, wounds, burns, and sprains, wherever soothing is needed.

I keep seeing the term "vulnerary" applied to St. John's Wort. What does it mean?

Herbs with this action are applied externally to promote swift healing of cuts and other punctures to the skin; the word's origins refer to the Latin term for wound.

If St. John's Wort is a styptic, will it reduce the bleeding from small cuts?

That's precisely what styptic means: an agent that helps slow or stop the flow of blood from minor cuts and punctures. It accomplishes this by acting as an astringent (see above).

Can it really help heal cuts?

The earliest folklore surrounding the herb mentions this use, and St. John's Wort has been used for over two millennia in the treatment of cuts and puncture wounds. Enough anecdotal evidence alone exists to support this claim strongly, but numerous tests have shown significant antibiotic actions in the herb. So you could consider that St. John's Wort has been scientifically proven to kill the bacteria and other microorganisms that could cause infections in wounds. In Germany, topical preparations of the herb are approved for labeling as treatments for wounds, although no studies have proven this to the standards of the FDA. Finally, there is some evidence that St. John's Wort also acts as a styptic, including a study where it reduced blood loss after an operation. The herb's astringent effects may help wounds, too, puckering the skin to reduce flow of blood from cuts.

To treat wounds with St. John's Wort, apply compresses doused in a wash of the herb, and continue to moisten dressings with it, or apply creams or oils made from St. John's Wort directly to the wound. Use this remedy only for relatively minor wounds, however. See your doctor if the wound is bleeding profusely, continues to bleed for a long period, if you experience numbness or tingling at the site, the wound is gaping too far for an adhesive bandage to seal, or is in an area where you don't want to run the risk of scarring.

Cuts on your fingers and hand run more risk of getting infected since they are constantly in contact with surfaces that may have bacteria—wash your hands frequently and see a doctor at the first sign of infection. Exercise even more caution with wounds on the face, chest, abdomen, or back, particularly punctures where the depth of the wound is hard to calculate. Wounds in those areas have more potential to reach vital organs and should be treated by a doctor unless they are very superficial. Puncture wounds over joints should be checked out by a doctor, too.

Medical assistance is definitely indicated if you develop a fever, pus begins to form, swelling persists, or if red streaks begin to form around the wound—these indicate the spread of infection. Remember, too, that tetanus shots only protect you from a potentially deadly infection of the nervous system for a period of about 10 years if you are an adult, and that children need a complete series of the shots to develop an immunity. If there's a chance you're not "covered," see your doctor about getting a booster. The brief moment of pain you may experience from the shot could save you a lot of grief that not even St. John's Wort could help!

Should you use St. John's Wort as a massage oil for sore muscles?

In Germany, the herb is a government-sanctioned therapy for muscle pain. Plenty of anecdotal accounts are traded regarding its ability to reduce the swelling associated with sore muscles, a result of the herb's anti-inflammatory effects. Both oil and cream preparations of the herb are used for this application.

I've heard people use St. John's Wort on sunburn—but also that skin burns are a side effect. Is either rumor true?

As an oil, cream or other form of balm, St. John's Wort has been used for over 2,000 years in the treatment of minor burns, including sunburn. Extensive anecdotal evidence exists, as well as studies on its antibacterial effects that strongly support this use. In Germany it is a medically accepted therapy for first-degree burns. (First-degree burns are categorized as those burns affecting just the topmost layer of skin, or epidermis, which produce only redness and some swelling—not blistering.) Even with all this evidence of successful use, stop applying the herb and see a doctor if the burn begins to produce pus, looks very red, or has an odd odor. That may mean the burn site has become infected.

The side effect of sunburn you have heard about as a symptom of St. John's Wort use is known as phototoxicity. Most of the alarms about this side effect of St. John's Wort stem from documented cases of this effect in cattle grazing on the herb, which is why it is sometimes called "hypericism." But these animals, which have reportedly included cows, lambs, and goats, were eating enormous amounts of the herb grown in sunny conditions (which increases hypericin content), were constantly exposed to strong sunlight while eating the herb, and have digestive systems very different from our own. Other mammals tested on the herb, even at high doses, did not experience this effect.

The only clinically documented cases of phototoxic effects from St. John's Wort use in humans arose from intravenous doses of synthesized hypericin, which were used in AIDS studies. A few anecdotal reports have also come in from people who took commercial preparations of whole-herb St. John's Wort in far higher doses than normal; most of these were HIV-infected patients unsuccessfully attempting to achieve the same concentrations of active ingredients used in antiviral clinical studies. If you take normal doses of the herb, your chances of getting burned seem minimal. To play it absolutely safe until further testing rules out phototoxicity for good, you may want to limit exposure to sun or wear a sunscreen while using the herb, especially if you have fair skin.

What about other skin conditions? Will St. John's Wort work on rashes or sores?

There are some anecdotal accounts of use on skin rashes, sores, and other skin eruptions. Obviously the herb's anti-inflammatory actions are important here, and its bacteria-fighting agents may also prevent the spread of infection. If you develop a fever or chills, or if the redness and swelling start to spread, discontinue use of the herb and see a doctor; an infection has probably set in. Other skin conditions that have been anecdotally treated with St. John's Wort include shingles and boils. Shingles is a late complication of chicken pox. The virus that causes the acute infection, varicella, is a member of the herpes family. After chicken pox, the virus may "reside" within sensory nerve cells as a latent or dormant infection. Later, especially during time of stress or illness, the viral infection erupts along the distribution of the infected nerve cells. Shingles is characterized by burning, itchy, and painful blisters, and usually runs a one- to two-week course without complications. Shingles should be treated by a doctor if the infection occurs near the eyes, as blindness could result if left untreated.

Boils are infections affecting hair follicles, and are also known as carbuncles and furuncles. These are funny-sounding terms for unpleasant conditions resulting in round, painful, pimplelike knobs filled with pus. Creams, oils, or washes of St. John's Wort have been reported as effective on these conditions, but you probably will get speedier relief if the boil is drained surgically and/or a potent antibiotic is prescribed.

My herbalist suggested I use St. John's Wort after I got a tooth yanked by the dentist. Is it safe?

I ran across a couple of recent articles in alternative-medicine newsletters touting this use of the herb, and a few homeopathic journals have also listed St. John's Wort as a remedy for toothache and relief of pain from an extraction or drilling. This effect is no doubt due to the herb's noted analgesic actions. As an anti-inflammatory it would also help reduce the swelling that often follows dental work. Because the herb is not toxic when taken internally in normal doses, it should be safe (provided you use applications made with edible ingredients—some creams would not be appropriate for internal use). Try drinking the tea for this therapy, or rubbing in a little of the oil-based extract. It may not taste good, but it shouldn't cause harm if you have learned you are not allergic to the herb. Just watch out for signs of infection—persistent pain, continued swelling and redness, or fever and chills.

I heard something about St. John's Wort being an antioxidant. Is there anything in it that targets free radicals?

There are a number of constituents of St. John's Wort that are suspected of having antioxidant properties, among them rutin and quercetin. However, the current flurry of rumors about St. John's Wort's antioxidant properties no doubt arose because the bioflavonoid procyanidin is one of its constituents. Unfortunately, procyanidin is present in the herb in only low levels. Remember, too, that the avalanche of ads and products currently touting procyanidins as an age-preventing, cancer-fighting, heart-enhancing, arthritis cures are just that—ads geared to separate you from your money. The claims they make about procyanidins, ranging from cures for AIDS, dry skin, jet lag, horse cancers, and multiple sclerosis, are still being studied and are far from definitive. In addition, these claims are made about compounds, or blends, which most often count grape seeds or pine bark as their prime nutrients, not St. John's Wort. Such compounds are known under the patented name Pycnogenol, a term sometimes used interchangeably (but mistakenly) with the single component procyanidin. In turn, procyanidin has the synonyms oligomeric proanthocyanidin, sometimes called OTCs, procyanidol and procyanidine. (There are lots of different kinds of procyanidins, too, like eicatechin 3-O-gallate, epigallocatechin 3-O-gallate, catechins, epicatechins, and flavon-3-O.)

Confused yet? Some companies are banking on that, and any that make claims about St. John's Wort targeting free radicals are taking advantage of the fact that you don't have a degree in chemistry. For the record:

- "Free radicals" is the term given to molecules that are missing electrons. Electrons circle molecules in much the way the moon orbits the Earth, except electrons prefer to travel in pairs. When one of a pair is missing, and the molecule is thus circled by an odd number of electrons, the molecule becomes a free radical. The incomplete molecule goes searching for its missing part (think of the headless horseman) and wrests electrons from other molecules, such as those found in cell membranes and DNA. These molecules then become free radicals which themselves attack other molecules and . . . you get the idea. This continuing chain reaction can damage hundreds, thousands, perhaps even a million cells throughout your body.

- Among other effects, the multiplying process of free radicals produces oxidation. Oxidation speeds decay of many organisms; it's the thing causing metal to rust, foods to spoil, and, in humans, it is implicated in the more apparent effects of aging—wrinkles and conditions like arthritis, heart disease, and cancer. Antioxidants, also known as free-radical scavengers, are elements that stop or slow this process. Some well-known natural antioxidants are the vitamins A, C, and E, also selenium and beta-carotene.

- A test was conducted in Russia that indicated some antioxidant action from St. John's Wort when used in combination with riboflavin. *Hypericum* rated the highest in efficiency as an antioxidant of the various plants tested. It was one very limited test, however, and simply compared St. John's Wort to other herbs like valerian and ginseng. Many more, well-documented studies would have to be performed before anyone could make claims that St. John's Wort scavenges free radicals.

- If you want to prevent the production of free radicals, St. John's Wort is not the answer. While it appears all bioflavonoids are, to some extent, antioxidants, to just what extent remains unclear. And even if the procyanidins in St. John's Wort have the same effect as those produced in pine bark and grape seeds, which is doubtful in the low concentration, oral ingestion does not seem to have an effect. Since intravenous dosing would be a difficult treatment option, you should instead avoid situations which expose you to environmental pollution such as smoky atmospheres, chlorofluorocarbons (CFCs), car emissions, or pest and weed killers. Too much exercise can generate increased free radical amounts, as can chemotherapy or X-rays. Stress and poor nutrition are contributing factors to free-radical production. Regularly take vitamin supplements containing antioxidant vitamins, or eat foods rich in them, like garlic and kale. But since oxygen and the laws of thermodynamics are the prime causes of free radicals, do not think you can eliminate them completely.

What's an adjuvant? I heard St. John's Wort described that way in an herbal mixture.

An herb is termed an adjuvant when it is included in a compound to help support the actions of another ingredient. For instance, St. John's Wort is often added to diet mixtures not because it will address the physical causes and results of weight gain, but because it may promote weight loss by helping to alleviate the depression that so often accompanies a weight problem.

I've heard St. John's Wort is the new Phen-Fen. Can it really help me lose weight?

Anecdotal reports that St. John's Wort may affect appetite pop up from time to time, but are few and far between. Nevertheless, the herb has been gaining an increasing reputation as a dieting "drug." Why? Probably because it is a common ingredient in the herbal alternatives to Phen-Fen, which started cropping up as soon as that chemical compound was yanked from shelves. Phen-Fen is a combination of two drugs, phentermine and fenfluramine, which were paired for treatment of extreme obesity. When the combination became more widely used, there were a number of severe reactions, and fenfluramine was withdrawn from the market. In addition, it has long been known that phentermine can be habit-forming and can cause serious psychiatric side effects, like hallucinations or marked mood swings.

To be blunt, there is no "natural Phen-Fen." This is, plain and simply, profiteering and deceptive advertising. The effects of St. John's Wort as a dieting aid are similarly suspect. Far more likely is that the herb's antidepressant effects are at play in these dieting compounds. By enhancing positive feelings, improving mood, and chipping away at the burden of minor depression, St. John's Wort may relieve some of the feelings of sadness and low self-esteem that drive people to eat excess amounts in the first place. These effects, while positive, do not really address the root causes of poor self-image and depression, so people who use food as a balm might also consider therapy for these other issues.

More importantly, though, dieting aids containing St. John's Wort as just one of several ingredients should be avoided *because* of those other ingredients. The use of *Ephedra* in many of these herbal Phen-Fen alternatives is arousing a great deal of concern at the FDA and among physicians. *Ephedra,* also known as Ma Huang, is a powerful herb with potentially dangerous stimulant effects on the heart and nervous system, like a potent caffeine. Hundreds of reports of adverse "events"— such as shortness of breath, rapid heartbeat, tremors, insomnia, and high blood pressure—have been made to the FDA and other agencies in relation to use of products containing epherine alkaloid-producing ingredients like *Ephedra.* Strokes, heart attacks, and even deaths have numbered among these reports.

These all gave rise to a recent warning from the FDA against dieting aids promoted as herbal Phen-Fens. As if the *Ephedra* connection weren't enough, some of these mixtures also include 5-hydroxytryptophan, a compound closely related to L-tryptophan. L-tryptophan is the dietary precursor of serotonin that was notoriously removed from the U.S. market in 1990 when it was discovered that product impurities caused a blood disorder involved in over 1,000 deaths. I would urge extreme caution in the use of any herbal dieting aid. Most of these are mixtures that, even if they don't contain the ingredients noted here, have never been tested in combination with each other. Mixtures like that are always riskier than therapies using a single ingredient.

And if that isn't reason enough here's one more—so far there is absolutely *no* evidence these even work on appetite control, not even anecdotal reports. So dieters are running quite a risk.

I don't have depression, but I'm currently taking Elavil for fibromyalgia. Can I switch to St. John's Wort?

A disorder that affects the musculoskeletal system, fibromyalgia is similar to rheumatoid arthritis, but has a greater impact on the body's fiberlike connective tissues. It may produce flulike symptoms including fatigue, in addition to chronic arthritis-like pain. Fibromyalgia is a relatively newly recognized condition that remains difficult to diagnose; it is mainly identified when a patient responds with pain when pressure is applied to a number of trigger points around the body. Depression is a common partner to this disorder, almost inextricably intertwined with fatigue and chronic pain.

So it is perhaps not surprising that a number of fibromyalgia sufferers have traded anecdotal accounts of relief with treatment of St. John's Wort. The herb may have anti-inflammatory actions on the condition, but almost certainly works as an antidepressant, making the symptoms of fibromyalgia a little easier to live with. Treatments for the pain of fibromyalgia have not yet been defined; many people with this condition are using prescription antidepressants like Elavil to help them cope with the constant ache. Use of St. John's Wort in this case seems like a viable alternative that warrants closer study. Check with your doctor to see if the herb is indicated, and to discuss the consequences of being withdrawn from current medications in order to use St. John's Wort.

Fibromyalgia is sometimes associated with chronic fatigue syndrome and Epstein-Barr virus, which also may benefit from treatment with St. John's Wort. See more about the herb's antiviral effects below.

I've heard St. John's Wort may work on Epstein-Barr. Any truth to the rumor?

Studies exist showing the herb has an effect on Epstein-Barr virus (also known as EBV), which causes mononucleosis and may be implicated in more extended bouts of persistent fatigue. Epstein-Barr is only one of several viruses observed in studies of chronic fatigue syndrome and has not been the focus of its own test. The extent of these studies on human subjects is not such that would make it a definitive treatment for the condition. But they certainly support the overall classification of St. John's Wort, and particularly hypericin and pseudohypericin, as possible antiviral medications. More importantly, many people with chronic fatigue syndrome obtain some relief from nonsedating or "energizing" antidepressants, and St. John's Wort certainly is used for this purpose.

What effect does the herb have on tuberculosis?

Studies on the herb's actions against *Mycobacterium tuberculosis* have been promising, but keep in mind that these studies were performed on the tuberculosis microbes in test tubes, not on human subjects. In these tests, extracts of St. John's Wort inhibited the growth of bacteria—it had similar effects on other bacteria tested, including staphylococci (infectious bacteria that infects the skin or strike the throat and lungs as a type of pneumonia), shigella (a bacterium producing gastroenteritis and dysentery), and *Escherichia coli* (a species of bacteria that is frequently the culprit behind infections of wounds and in the urinary tract). There are other treatments for these conditions you should consider; until we know more about the herb's antibacterial effect in humans, consult with your doctor to see if St. John's Wort is really the best option.

Is St. John's Wort a cure for leukemia?

It is very unlikely that St. John's Wort will be found to be a cure for leukemia. There are very preliminary data on the subject that are encouraging, however, that St. John's Wort may help. A study was conducted in 1988 testing hypericin on mice that had been infected with Friend leukemia and radiation leukemia viruses. Results indicated that St. John's Wort helped the infected mice to live longer, and even stopped the disease from spreading to new cells. Will it have the same effect on the types of leukemia that afflict people? It's too early to tell. If you or a loved one have leukemia, talk with your doctor about the pros and cons of taking St. John's Wort in addition to your standard medications.

What can St. John's Wort do for viruses like the flu?

The same studies conducted on leukemia also involved a strain of influenza and the herb had similar impact on the influenza virus—stopping infection of new cells. That holds promise for its treatment of this recurrent visitor, a promise confirming the anecdotal evidence which has collected for years of the herb's effects on colds and flu. (Remember, flu is distinguished from colds by severity of symptoms, aches and pains, chills, and presence of a fever.) St. John's Wort's suspected antiviral activities might have the potential to slow or halt progression of flu once a person has been infected, but in the meantime, the herb's other potential actions (analgesic, expectorant, anti-inflammatory) could help alleviate the symptoms which do present, like the miscellaneous aches, congestion, coughs, and sore throats common to these viral infections. Concrete evidence is still far away, but since mild cases of flu are routinely treated by a host of alternative or folk medicines—from St. John's Wort to chicken soup—use of St. John's Wort seems relatively harmless, as long as you also get bed rest and drink plenty of fluids. But be aware of how the virus affects you and be alert for anything that may set this bout of flu apart: If it seems especially long-lived, you are already run-down and fatigued when it strikes, you experience trouble breathing, you feel confused or especially lethargic, your neck feels stiff, a rash appears, vomiting persists, or your fever passes 102 degrees, see a doctor *right away*. Some strains of influenza can still be fatal when they lead to a bacterial pneumonia or, in people already weakened by fatigue or other conditions, a complete shutdown of body functions could occur, resulting in death. Also, even if you find that St. John's Wort helps lessen the symptoms of a viral infection, you should not overlook the value of annual flu shots to prevent the illness.

I've been diagnosed with herpes simplex. I would really love to self-treat it, so no one will know. Can St. John's Wort help?

As with any disease, you should never self-treat without a diagnosis by a doctor and a discussion about how each therapy would interact with your unique expression of the illness. I assume here that you are talking about herpes simplex type 2 rather than type 1 infection that causes "cold sores" and "fever blisters." Fortunately, unless you make a general announcement to friends and coworkers, no one will know why you are seeing your physician. If you're concerned about telling a doctor, believe me, they see such a variety of illnesses and people that it usually does not occur to them to make judgments about something as common as herpes. Painful and embarrassing as this illness may be for you, it's all in a day's work for a physician. Doctors know that people have sex and that, because genital herpes infections are only episodically symptomatic, that you probably had no idea what you were getting into. If your current doctor makes you feel uncomfortable about your condition, look for another one. That is simply not the right caregiver for you. However, if you and your doctor determine that St. John's Wort is a safe road to follow, there are anecdotal reports that it may be helpful when used topically (i.e., applied directly to the herpes blisters).

Studies show some action against strains of herpes simplex virus (HSV-1 and HSV-2) when the herb is used against the virus in *in vitro,* or test-tube, studies. That last bit of information is very important, because it means these studies were not conducted on human subjects (which are known as *in vivo* studies). So whether the herb will work for you and your herpes infection is not at all clear. On the bright side, it was the success of St. John's Wort in the treatment of herpes simplex, influenza, and other viruses that first attracted the attention of the researchers studying its use against AIDS. They felt since St. John's Wort seemed to be effective against those viruses, perhaps it could have similar actions against other viral-based illnesses. Keep in mind that the *in vitro* trials of St. John's Wort on herpes simplex were not extensive, and no definitive studies have been conducted on humans, so it's still anybody's guess on whether it is truly effective in the long run. Try other, more established treatments for your herpes before attempting to self-treat with a remedy that is so uncertain.

What's going on with AIDS-HIV testing of the drug? I've heard only rumors about it.

Hypericin, one of the chemical components of St. John's Wort, continues to be tested for use in the treatment of Acquired Immune Deficiency Syndrome (AIDS). Recent reports from the International Conference on AIDS, published in the *British Medical Journal,* tracked patients infected with HIV (*human immunodeficiency virus*) over a period of forty months. The tests were conducted under the auspices of the National Institute for Allergies and Infectious Diseases, a division of the National Institutes of Health (NIH), which sponsored the studies. In laymen's terms, these trials noted the following:

1. Hypericin inhibits or slows all stages of the virus's process of infection. These include binding and entry (when

a virus combines with a healthy cell), reverse transcriptase (production of a viral enzyme), transcription and translation (exchange of infection), and maturation and budding (a separate, newly infected cell)—but especially the crucial early stages. Hypericin seemed to bind with the membranes of the HIV virus, and this action in some way slowed or prevented the virus from infecting new cells. Apparently hypericin interacts with oxygen in a process that prevents the virus cells from "uncoating," or stripping off, their outer protein shells. That would make it more difficult, perhaps impossible, for the virus to infect healthy cells.

2. As what's called a "broad-spectrum virucidal agent," hypericin acts on a whole range of infectious microorganisms and may attack the AIDS virus in a different way than other medications currently used to treat the disease. Therefore, it could be used in combination with the other drugs for a two-pronged attack on the virus, without multiplying the risk of side effects by overdosing, and could be helpful treating people unable to tolerate those other forms of therapy.

To obtain these results, 18 HIV-infected patients were observed from four to six years, under treatment with plant-derived extracts of St. John's Wort. The extracts, supplied by a company called VIMRX, were taken both intravenously and in tablet form. Of these patients:

- Thirty-three percent had concentrations of serum p24 antigen (a hallmark of the activity of HIV infection) present in their bodies prior to receiving treatment with St. John's Wort. Of those patients, only one became HIV-positive during the initial twenty-four months of the study; all the others remained negative during the study and throughout post-treatment follow-ups.
- Four of the six volunteers with the antigen showed a decline in levels during the trial. In the other two people, levels remained stable.
- The viral load in most of these patients declined, even if they were p24 antigen–positive. In those patients whose viral load increased, no corresponding clinical complica-

tions occurred—usually there are clinical symptoms that accompany any such rise.

An earlier report on the same study gave some additional information:

- The values for helper T cells remained stable or rose during the forty-month trial. Levels of leukocytes, hemoglobin, and platelets also remained the same.
- Only two of the sixteen people in the study experienced some type of infection during the study; the others remained infection-free. This is a surprisingly low rate. Typically, AIDS sufferers are vulnerable to a variety of other viruses, such as leukemia. In fact, no cases of complications involving herpes, Epstein-Barr virus, and cytomegalovirus were encountered by any of the patients.
- None of the phototoxic side effects that plagued earlier trials was experienced. In fact, no side effects of note were reported at all.

What can an herb do to help treat something as serious as AIDS?

First, remember that researchers have been testing the use of concentrated extracts of hypericin and pseudohypericin, two of the many "ingredients" in St. John's Wort rather than extracts of the whole *Hypericum perforatum* plant, which is what you can buy in stores. Some even used extracts from a different species from the same herb family, called *Hypericum triquetrifolium*. As for its use in AIDS therapy—tests indicate that hypericin works as an "antiretroviral." Simply put, it appears to inhibit the spread of the viruses. It may achieve this effect by making it more difficult for HIV to penetrate and infect healthy cells, by blocking its capacity to form the abnormally large cells that may spread the virus, or by inactivating the virus itself. But most of these are just theories about the effects of hypericin on AIDS, derived from observing the herb's effects on viruses in the test tube. One test published in the *British Medical Journal* noted immunotropic or immune-boosting properties in St. John's Wort, possibly a result of the herb's polyphenol ingredients. Still, exactly how the herb may work against retroviruses is unclear. But when tested in animal studies on viruses similar to AIDS, hypericin caused the virus to become inactive and appeared to check the infection of new cells.

What were the results of the early tests of retroviruses?

In 1988 a team of researchers at New York University led by Dr. Daniel Muruelo published the results of their first studies on mice, a subject that was also on the agenda at the meeting of the National Academy of Sciences that same year. Because there is no instance of HIV infection in mice, St. John's Wort was tested on a retrovirus that has similar effects on rodents, a strain of Friend leukemia. Results were very encouraging: after just one dose of the herbal extract, spread of the disease was slowed or stopped in a majority of the mice tested. These mice typically live for only twenty-five days when exposed to the virus, and no mice in the control group survived past that marker, but almost half the rodents treated with St. John's Wort lived for the duration of the study—a full 150 days. (Some reports place the survival rate at even longer for some of the mice, up to 240 days.) Moreover, all of the untreated mice developed an enlarged spleen, whereas none of those treated with St. John's Wort developed this complication. Also promising was the fact that the mice experienced few noticeable side effects.

These same studies showed another surprising result—St. John's Wort does not appear to work in the same way as other HIV treatments like AZT, which affect levels of reverse transcriptase, an enzyme in the body. In fact, these limited clinical studies showed that low doses of both herb and AZT were effective when used in combination, but that these doses have little or no impact when used separately. That may indicate a possibility of using the herb in combination with those other medications, creating a ''one-two'' punch against the virus, at lower doses of AZT that may not produce the toxic side effects so prevalent with that drug. Remember, though, that all of this information is extremely preliminary—many more studies are needed to support these initial results—and, of course, these were performed on mice, not humans.

I heard that the human testing had been stopped because of bad side effects.

After the early tests on mice, trials were quickly scheduled on human subjects—patients already infected with HIV. These subjects were divided into groups; some took concentrated extracts of St. John's Wort orally, others were given various doses of a chemically synthesized (man-made) hypericin extract, taken intravenously. This first cycle of human trials in the early nineties was, indeed, stopped before it was completed—too many of the volunteers given the synthesized hypericin experienced extreme phototoxic side effects, receiving bad burns when exposed to sunlight. Researchers and the company that created the synthesized hypericin, VIMRX, went back to the drawing board, in order to produce a synthesized version of hypericin that could be administered by mouth (since subjects receiving it orally did not experience the same side effects as those who received it intravenously), or at lower doses that would be taken intravenously more frequently. The most recent human trials that concluded in 1996 used this newer version of the medication. Obviously, the combination used succeeded in this goal, as no phototoxic effects were documented and the study was completed with no problems.

Have there been other studies on human subjects?

A few doctors aware of the early tests of St. John's Wort on infected rodents or the first, aborted trial on human subjects immediately began performing less formal testing on volunteer patients who were HIV-positive. Most of these informal studies did not use the concentrated doses that seemed indicated by the testing on mice, but utilized more commonly available versions of the plant extract (teas, low-dose tablets, or the standardized forms of the herb sold as antidepressants in Germany, such as Hyperforat or LI-160). Sure enough, the results of these scattered tests have been less positive even though such informal studies tend to yield more inflated results. While many of the patients reportedly experienced significant alleviation of symptoms of the infection, including mood improvement, higher levels of energy, and better appetite, these could all be related to the antidepressant actions of the herb rather than any antiviral effects. Change in T-cell counts and spread of the disease were not affected by these standard doses of St. John's Wort. It appears higher levels of hypericin and pseudohypericin are required to have a significant effect on HIV.

Even more informally, a tiny number of patients who have

been unable to tolerate more traditional AIDS-HIV "cocktails" are conducting their own tests under the supervision of their individual physicians—some of whom have been in contact with the team at NYU Medical Center for advice. Somewhat dated anecdotal evidence from these patients also shows no noticeable increase in T-cell counts, but the medication had a marked impact on other symptoms, such as pain, nausea, fatigue, and sleeplessness. This marked improvement occurred only in those taking extracts of the herb; patients using teas with largely unknown quantities of hypericin experienced far fewer benefits and more side effects. It should be noted, however, that this information is completely anecdotal, no focused long-term follow-up has been conducted, and these patients were using a wide range of preparations of St. John's Wort, sometimes at unusually high dosages.

I am HIV-positive *now*. I can't wait 10 years to see the results of testing. Is St. John's Wort safe to use now, just in case it does work?

Safe? Probably, if you use standard doses under the care of a physician who's already treating you for the disease and is familiar with possible interactions with other medications in your therapy plan.

Effective? That's what the testing hopes to prove, and the best intentions in the world won't make it go faster than the nature of clinical research on this complex illness allows. In the meantime, I know of patients who attempted to achieve higher concentrations of hypericin and pseudohypericin by simply taking larger doses of commercial extracts, or drinking many, many cups of tea, and apparently experienced side effects that made continued treatment impossible—burns from sun exposure and debilitating nausea. All of these factors should indicate caution for even the most desperate person with the idea of self-treating with this herb.

Even if St. John's Wort or its constituent hypericin is eventually proven effective in the treatment of AIDS—not definitively shown yet by any means—anecdotal evidence strongly suggests that dosing yourself with enough of commercial preparations to mimic the amounts of hypericin used in clinical testing also greatly increases the likelihood of side effects. The long-term effects of such high dosages is unknown, too. We can't use safety statistics based on the decades-long use of St. John's Wort in Germany, either, since the amount used in depression treatment is nowhere near as high as that being tested for AIDS.

Are you sure I can't just multiply the normal doses of St. John's Wort?

Even the doctors conducting early trials on St. John's Wort and AIDS have expressed concern that the success of those tests will induce people infected with HIV to overdose in their attempts to use the herb as a treatment. They feel that commercial preparations *simply will not* supply the necessary amounts of hypericin, and that hopes may be raised only to be crushed when standard doses of the herb prove ineffective. The options for treatment of HIV-positive patients are better now than ever; I would strongly recommend exploring them before committing yourself to a treatment that might turn out to be ineffective or even dangerous. If those other options have been exhausted by you and your treatment team, bring the information about St. John's Wort to your physician, so together you can make a knowledgeable decision. If your condition warrants an immediate look at hypericin, consider volunteering for any new trials at your local research hospital, so your experimentation can be done under appropriate medical supervision.

Will it really work on cancer? It would be a miracle.

The National Cancer Institute is sponsoring some tests on the use of St. John's Wort in the treatment of cancer, following earlier studies that showed promising antitumor and antimutagenic action on cancer in rodents and photodynamic effects in test-tube studies. But before you get too excited, you should know that the National Cancer Institute screens about 10,000 plants a year for effects on cancer—after twenty-five years and about 114,000 plants only 4% have shown anticancer actions that could be reproduced in studies. Also know that some of the studies on hamsters did not show any such anticancer action. Obviously, a lot more work needs to be done to find out the true antimutagenic effect on this action of the herb.

In the meantime, though, here's what those promising preliminary studies have shown:

- Some of St. John's Wort potential effects on cancer can be traced to the antioxidant actions performed by several of the herb's constituents.
- Antineoplastic properties seem indicated. This means the herb (or some of its constituents, like hypericin), would have the ability to control or kill cancer cells. In some studies photosensitized hypericin caused a complete inhibition of tumor growth.
- Rodents with cancers were able to maintain or even increase body weight when treated with the herb.
- The bioflavonoid quercetin, found in the herb, may have antimutagenic action. This would mean it could slow or stop the mutating of cells in the body. Mutated cells are responsible for a wide array of disorders, including cancer. A note of caution, however: One of the studies on hamsters showed no such effect. These results have generated some controversy, as cancer in hamsters is not as complex as cancer in humans. Clearly, more trials focusing on this action need to be conducted.

All of this sends some hopeful signals about the herb. But cancer sufferers have heard the siren call before and had their hopes crushed, so should exercise the same caution toward this therapy they do to others. The time needed to prove or disprove scientifically the herb's effects will render this treatment moot for many patients, unless they are willing to try experiments that could cost them time on another treatment. But if you're undergoing treatment for cancer and are interested in exploring this therapy, discuss the latest studies with your doctor; more may become known in the period since this book was written.

What does "photodynamic" or "photosensitized" mean in relation to cancer and antiviral therapy?

In antiviral studies, the chemical hypericin was also exposed to light, making its actions more powerful. As for cancer studies, recent testing indicates that cancerous cells bind with hypericin when a "patient" with cancer (read: rodent) has been exposed to radiation therapy. Once binding occurs, hypericin makes the cancerous cells even more susceptible than they normally are to the damaging rays of radiation. This is perhaps not surprising when you recall how the potency of hypericin in the herb St. John's Wort responds to exposure to sunlight. Not only that. It appears that healthy cells do not bind in the same way with the chemical. So what does that *really* mean? If further tests support those very preliminary results, it would mean that hypericin could be used to fine-tune the effects of radiation therapy—perhaps fewer or lower doses of harmful radiation would be necessary to kill off cancer cells if hypericin causes the mutated cells to react more intensely to the therapy. The harmful side effects of radiation therapy could be significantly reduced if that was the case, and recovery would be much speedier. In antiviral therapy, hypericin's actions are likewise heightened after it has been exposed to light or radiation.

Oddly, while exposure to radiation enhances hypericin's effects on cancer cells, a Russian test on St. John's Wort's ability to *protect* marrow and mucus of the thin intestine from the harmful effects of X-rays had some encouraging results when performed on mice. So it may be that St. John's Wort enhances the effects of chemotherapy on mutated cells while at the same time having radioprotective properties, protecting healthy cells. However, this was a single test performed on rodents, not humans—the potential is exciting, but neither one of these effects has been studied enough to draw any conclusions.

How is the herb taken for all these medical purposes?

St. John's Wort can be administered in any number of ways. Eating the raw plant is not advised, as its bitter flavor will pretty much guarantee you wouldn't eat enough to get any kind of medicinal benefit. It's not dangerous to do so, though, unless you are one of the rare people allergic to the herb—and you would never eat as many plants as would be necessary to generate the phototoxicity effects that have been noted in grazing cattle. Rather than eat the raw herb, you should choose one of the "processed" versions of the St. John's Wort, selected for its effectiveness in the application you require. "Standardized" extracts will ensure you get a certain amount of hypericin—whether it's enough to treat a specific condition or even the constituent that works on the condition for which you're taking the herb is another issue. If the procyanidins or bioflavonoids like quercetin are what you need, then you can only guess at the amounts you're getting, as these ingredients are not measured along with the hypericin.

The commercial preparations include: infusions, such as teas, made from the dried herb; extracts of the macerated (shredded) herb soaked in alcohol or glycerin; oils made from a similar soaking done in vegetable oil; ointments; or capsules, tablets and pills made from powdered St. John's Wort. (See more guidelines on the various preparations in Chapters Seven and Eight, and in the individual entries above.)

If St. John's Wort has "medicinal" effects on so many conditions, doesn't that mean it's a drug?

Currently, St. John's Wort is classified as a dietary supplement in the United States, even though it has been approved as a treatment for depression, wounds, first-degree burns, and muscle pain in some foreign countries, notably Germany. Still, very limited testing has been done on most of the other actions ascribed to the herb—nothing like the extent of scrutiny it has received for depression and is now getting for cancer and viruses like AIDS—and so I wouldn't look for the FDA to approve many of those other uses anytime soon.

In order to clarify its role as a therapeutic, though, St. John's Wort is sometimes described under terms other than dietary supplement. These terms, "phytomedicines" and "neutricicals," were coined by individuals for plant-based treatments. Phytomedicines are defined as therapies derived solely from plants—no other ingredients are found in these compounds. They may consist of the whole plant or extracts derived from plant material. The term was first introduced by a French doctor, Henri Leclerc, in the early twentieth century. It's only recently become popularly used, however, as interest in herbal remedies returns to something like the levels it enjoyed prior to this century. Remember, though, that the evidence suggesting the herb is effective for many of the uses for which it is credited may be very limited or even purely anecdotal. Using it for any of the conditions noted may be a risk on one level or another. Further research on your part will ensure that it's a risk you have calculated carefully.

What's the weirdest thing this herb can do?

I'd have to say its anecdotal use as an antidote for snakebites ranks up there. The herb has been noted with that action in Brazilian herbal lore and also by Native Americans after the herb was introduced in the U.S. Whether I would recommend dosing with the herb instead of running to the nearest hospital for antivenom is quite another issue. This is certainly one case where I'd stick with the more tried-and-true methods of treatment.

SEVEN

What You Should Know about Buying St. John's Wort or Other Herbal Remedies

Danny came into his doctor's office carrying a bottle of tablets in his hand. He had been using St. John's Wort for over a month, he reported, and had noticed no effect whatsoever—even though two of his friends suffering from similar cases of major depression had reported "incredible" success. Danny's doctor told him that every medicine has the potential to work differently for different people. Then the doctor took a look at the bottle; he wanted to read the fine print carefully to see whether the herbal preparation was standardized to include certain levels of active chemical agents. But there wasn't any fine print. Instead, in big, bold letters, the manufacturer made vague claims about "improving emotional balance." As a medical doctor familiar with the exhaustive entries on every brand of medicine in physician's desk references, Danny's doctor found the complete lack of basic information alarming. Then Danny pointed out that even when he gets prescriptions filled, they generally come with little or no information on the bottle either—except for a small sticker listing the name of the drug and how often to take it. "Mostly I just trust that one of us knows what we're doing—and it isn't me!" He laughed. After talking about ways Danny could find out more about the drugs he is pre-

234

scribed, the conversation turned back to St. John's Wort. Since neither Danny nor his doctor knew anything about this particular brand Danny had been taking, to trust it seemed misplaced. Danny's doctor recommended a brand he knew contained a formula used in clinical studies abroad. It seemed the most well-documented and reputable option, and was also easily available in local stores. Danny bought a bottle of the brand his doctor recommended and tried St. John's Wort again. However, he still had no significant changes to report at his next appointment. In the end, Danny decided St. John's Wort was not for him, even though his two friends continued to get relief with their herbal treatments. The good news: At least Danny knew it was his unique chemistry interacting with the herb and not simply a case of a bad brand.

Are there any "rules" for buying St. John's Wort?

The first rule, of course, is to make sure St. John's Wort is appropriate for treating what ails you. If your condition has not been diagnosed and treated by a professional—I strongly recommend you see to that first. Once you're certain what you're combating, read the chapters on depression and the use of St. John's Wort and consult your doctor, to help you determine whether you should be using this herb at all.

If you and your doctor decide that you should give St. John's Wort a try, then there are certainly some general rules to keep in mind:

Choose a brand that you trust. Look for the terms "standardized," "standardized extract," or simply "standard" applied to the hypericin content in any commercial preparation. Sadly, even this is not a perfect indicator, since no independent agency is currently testing commercial preparations to confirm they're truly what they say they are. Still, "standardization" is a good place to start.

Generally, you should stay away from any herbal mixtures—products that include more than one herb, or St. John's Wort in combination with other ingredients. There have been very few studies done on how various herbs interact, and even herbalists tend to shun mixtures, preferring to dose with one herb at a time. The clinical trials done on St. John's Wort have been performed with extracts of the herb, unmixed with other herbs.

Another buying tip is to be familiar with the Latin name for St. John's Wort (*Hypericum perforatum L.*, often shortened to *Hypericum perforatum*, or *H. perforatum*). For that matter, knowing the Latin botanical name of any herb or plant you're using for medicinal purposes is always a good idea. Common names for herbs are often used for the sake of convenience and instant "recognizability"—this book being a case in point—but when purchasing, always look for the Latin to be sure you're getting exactly what you need. Too many plants and herbs have different species within their families that may not have the same actions when used medicinally. *H. perforatum* is the species of *Hypericum* most often tested for use in treating depression. Others in the *Hypericum* family may not have the same levels of ingredients that seem indicated for this condition. Which leads to the final rule:

Read all labels carefully! Look for the key words noted above. And follow printed directions for dosages, cross-checking them against the recommendations given in Chapter 5.

I've purchased different brands of St. John's Wort from three different stores. Some seem to work better than others. Isn't it all the same?

Your body is a pretty accurate barometer in this case. As it turns out, not all batches of an herb are created equal. The variable combination of soil quality, rainfall, growing conditions, amount of sunlight, local contaminants, harvesting methods, and preparation—not to mention the unique "genetics" of each particular strain of the herb—all make for a pretty wide range of potencies. This is easier to understand when you think about the interest that wine lovers show when a new Beaujolais is introduced—will it be as good this year as last? Which region will produce the best this season? How will age affect its quality? Just as the grapes grown in one area may produce a better-tasting wine than a crop grown on the vineyard just a few miles away, so too can St. John's Wort vary from one area to the next, one year to the next. So don't look for strict equivalencies from brand to brand. This is an important difference between manufactured medications (a milligram of one brand weighs the same as a milligram of another). Despite the most sincere efforts of a manufacturer, there may be different amounts of active ingredients in every batch harvested. The only way to pinpoint its precise level of hypericin is to perform standardization tests on every batch made. Until that's done and criteria agreed on across the board, there may be different amounts of hypericin in one manufacturer's product than in another's, in individual bottles produced by the same manufacturer, or even between any pair of capsules within any single bottle. Given the wide range of variables, it's best to stick with the same brand throughout your treatment with St. John's Wort. Switch only if it's not working for you and your doctor suggests experimenting with another brand.

Is there any danger in getting all these varied levels of active ingredients?

Fortunately, even if one batch of the herb is more potent than another, no one ingredient, or constituent, of St. John's Wort is likely to be present in toxic amounts. As long as you follow dosing directions, you won't be at significantly more risk for side effects. Whether you're getting all the active ingredient you need is another question. The only real danger here is that you might be wasting time (and money) that could be better spent on a more effective treatment.

What does "standardization" mean anyway?

"Standardization" means the herb has been processed in a manner that controls how much of a single active ingredient makes it into an individual dose. With strict standardization, every batch is tested to see what levels they contain. In a perfect world, seeing that term on a label should mean that the manufacturer has performed certain measurement techniques, such as High Performance Liquid Chromatography (HPLC), to confirm that every capsule in every bottle contains precisely the same amount of the active ingredient. Herbal remedies containing true standardized extracts may cost more than other brands, but the cliché is true—"you get what you pay for."

So, does "standardization" mean the quality is guaranteed?

In the realm of herbal treatment, there are no real quality-control standards beyond the "satisfaction guaranteed" offers made by some of the more reputable companies. In those cases, you are being given the opportunity to be reimbursed for the cost of the herb if you didn't like the way it performed. Here in the U.S., herbs are considered dietary supplements, which means companies are not *required* to perform any standardization tests or offer any quality guarantees as they must with those substances classified as medicinal drugs. Companies are only held legally responsible for content if they make certain specific claims—for instance, if their packaging plainly states the ingredients contain 0.3% hypericin, they are legally liable to provide that content. But if they don't state the level of ingredients, they're under no obligation to provide more than a tiny trace of whatever product is being touted. And, unfortunately, even if a label reads "standardized to contain 0.3%" it doesn't mean that amount of hypericin is really in there. Stick with well-known, reputable brands that have more to lose if they become the target of an investigation. They'll typically have more incentive to make good on all their claims. Remember, since St. John's Wort is not regulated, no one is consistently checking up to see if *any* of these ingredient claims and hypericin levels are accurate.

Give me a break. You mean, even if a label says it's got 0.3% hypericin, I can't necessarily trust it?

Most of the herbal medications available in the U.S. have never been tested by independent authorities to be sure the content truly has undergone these standardization processes and that the active ingredient is indeed present in the amount stated. The FDA doesn't have the resources to test randomly every such product on the market—and the burden of proof is on the manufacturer. Manufacturers know this all too well, and the more unscrupulous take advantage of the fact. Recently, there was a scare in Los Angeles surrounding the use of the herb kava, when 50 people had to be hospitalized after using a product called fX Rush. The product listed kava (a "natural" stimulant) as its main ingredient, raising concerns over the herb's safety. But when police seized samples of the product, analysis revealed much higher levels of caffeine and a central nervous system depressant in the mix—neither of which was mentioned on the packaging. It turned out the toxic reaction wasn't the result of kava. People's fears about the herb were calmed—but the incident raised the larger and even more disturbing issue of inaccurate labeling. The product's manufacturer, Biolife Bioproducts, was sent a letter of warning by the FDA and is facing lawsuits. There are undoubtedly other companies misrepresenting their products as well.

Why aren't herbal remedies regulated? Is the government against natural remedies for some reason?

Some people in the pharmaceutical industry would be ecstatic if their medications were so neglected! As has been mentioned before, herbs fall into the fuzzy gray area known as dietary supplements, a category not strictly defined. After all, "dietary supplement" is not a very precise term, meaning literally "something added to the diet." Virtually anything you ingest could fall under that broad terminology, and herbs are only one of a number of food or nutritional items that do. The idea behind placing herbal remedies in this classification was not really a bad one: If the government classified herbals as drugs, the herbs would first have to undergo rigorous and very costly testing to meet federal criteria for safety and effectiveness. The government does not generally foot the bill for this process; pharmaceutical companies usually step up to the plate when a new medicine is being considered. But the FDA well knows that pharmaceutical companies will not financially sponsor testing for natural products, because they are not able to patent an herb. It is through ownership of a product that a company makes its money. Moreover, scientists often have had trouble identifying and synthesizing the active ingredients in St. John's Wort into a product that could be patented. So, think about it—if sponsored testing of the raw herb St. John's Wort proved successful, *any* company could produce its own brand of herbal remedy and some people would grow it at home. What kind of return would the sponsoring pharmaceutical company get if that happened? More than likely, some companies would be losing money as patients substituted the herb for some already synthesized and patented drug. For this reason, little funding is made available for testing herbal remedies. And if herbals were classified as "medicines" or "drugs" under current laws, they could not be sold until they were tested as safe and effective.

For many years, herbal remedies were *not* allowed to be sold in the States. The government regulators responded to that quandary in 1994 by creating the Dietary Supplement Health & Education Act (DSHEA), which classified herbals as food supplements, freeing them from the burden of testing and allowing them to become widely available. There is a cost for that freedom, however. Because they are not subject to the same stringent tests required of drugs, herbal remedies are not regulated and quality is not controlled to the same degree as synthetic drugs—in fact, it is not really controlled at all.

So now we have health product companies, which perhaps don't have the best reputations for quality control to begin with and who aren't heavily capitalized for testing, producing herbal therapies. And bingo—there's St. John's Wort. Fortunately, though, government regulators are becoming more aware of consumer interest in herbal remedies and the desire to have them regulated and standardized to some degree. Contrary to the opinion of some alternative-medicine advocates, there is not a conspiracy to prevent people from having access to these products behind their somewhat slow response. "Big government" and the "evil empires" of the pharmaceutical industry do not conspire. It's simply a question of finances. Do people want medical testing of alternative treatments more than they want money spent on education, law enforcement, or social services? Increasingly, the answer seems to be yes, at least to some degree, because we are seeing more money being spent now by government agencies on studies of these therapies, St. John's Wort among them. Witness the ongoing study being performed under the auspices of the National Institute for Mental Health, which may result in a reclassification of St. John's Wort as something more than simply a "dietary supplement."

If St. John's Wort isn't regulated, how can I know if the brand I buy is any good?

Unless you obtain documented proof from an independent agency that a particular brand is being standardized (no easy task), it's largely a matter of trust: You have to trust your doctor or some other expert, like a herbalist, to give you knowledgeable opinions. Or you must trust the people working in your local health-food store to give you good advice—if for no other reason than that you've made it clear you'll be back for more if the brand they suggest really works. Or you can trust an organization like a botanical society or an herbal association's recommendation, on the theory that they'll represent the best of their field and steer you away from poor examples of the trade. Or you must trust your own body to tell you: Is it working? Do you feel better? If the answer is yes, then it's a pretty good bet you've made the right choice.

I switched to a new brand that makes the same "standardized" claims as the old one I was using, but it doesn't seem to be working—and it makes me feel sick. What should I do?

First of all, you should stop taking it. If your doctor agrees that the side effects you're experiencing aren't severe or threatening enough to justify stopping this treatment altogether, switch back to your old brand and see whether the symptoms continue. If the problem is corrected by switching brands, then it's likely that the newer brand has quality-control problems. However, it may be that the effectiveness of St. John's Wort has run its course in your case, or that long-term use is resulting in more noticeable side effects. Because there hasn't been a definitive long-term study made on St. John's Wort we're not sure how your body may respond to even standardized doses over an extended period of time. If experimenting makes it clear there was something wrong with the other brand you were using, you and your doctor should submit a complaint to the FDA. The agency can't investigate every complaint they receive, or yank a product off the shelves unless there is documented proof of a connection between adverse reactions and a particular ingredient or brand. However, if they receive a number of complaints targeting a specific product, they will check into it and perhaps discover the company was making false claims about the ingredients.

I don't know how to read the product labels for the teas and capsules I've found. What does "0.3% from 300 mg," "90c" or "4:1" mean anyway?

In early 1997 the FDA proposed a series of changes to the packaging of over-the-counter drugs. These included the use

of more understandable language rather than technical lingo—
"lung" instead of "pulmonary" and the like. It would also
require clearer presentation of warnings and may make deci-
phering ingredient levels less confusing. It's felt this new rule
will impact on dietary supplements, too. For now, though, be
encouraged that "0.3% from 300mg" is just the information
you want to see on a label for St. John's Wort, providing it's
followed by the term "standardized" or "standardized extract." It means that 300 milligrams of the whole harvested
herb has yielded 0.3% hypericin content. That is the level of
hypericin used in many of the clinical trials performed on the
herb's effectiveness as a treatment for depression. The ratio
you noted, "4:1," refers to the proportion of raw herb to base
in an extract, for example four parts of the herb to one part
alcohol or glycerin. Don't be misled into thinking it's the ratio
of herb to active ingredient, which is more like 300:1. Finally,
"90c" could mean a count of 90 capsules in the package. Or
you might have misread the quantity "90cc," which means
90 cubic centimeters; in apothecary measurements, one cc of
water (or one milliliter) weighs one gram. You'll find a chart
of more such measurements in the next chapter, as well as
some common U.S. customary system/metric equivalents.

What could a company do to a natural remedy like St. John's Wort to make it "bad"?

Dietary supplements aren't strictly regulated. That leaves a
number of openings for a good herb to turn bad. The FDA
warns that problems can occur when:

- there are varying degrees of potency and concentration of
  active ingredients
- "foreign" substances are introduced into the product by
  accident (that's coy FDA-speak for everything from bits
  of neighboring plants to stray animal parts and fecal matter)
- contamination occurs after a product has shipped; perhaps
  it has been stored incorrectly or shelves have been stocked
  with old merchandise—for that reason you should never
  buy food or dietary supplement products from deep-
  discount shops like the popular "dollar" stores

- products are mislabeled, leading to confusion over their use, dosing, or even identity
- the supplement is not used correctly by the consumer or distributor

Any of these might lead to a bad reaction to even a relatively low-risk herb like St. John's Wort. Choosing a reputable brand and carefully studying the label can avoid some of these problems, however.

I saw a box of St. John's Wort capsules that said the herb could cure anything from depression to black eyes to cancer. How can they make claims like that?

Since their therapeutic effects do not have to be proven to the scientific standards of the FDA, dietary supplements are under government mandate not to make any claims regarding your health, mental or physical. Still, claims of varying kinds are often made, and it's often hard to call manufacturers on their promises when even the experts continue to debate the fine line between phrases like "prevents heart disease" and "lowers risk of heart disease." A clever turn of phrase can skirt the rules but still mislead consumers.

The confusion and lack of policing allow loopholes for manufacturers to exploit. And they take full advantage of it. A recent scan of commercial sites on the Internet revealed web-site ads for St. John's Wort labeled with any number of boasts, ranging from those couched in historical terms ("a flowering herb that has long been used to fight anxiety") to the vaguely promising ("popular for replenishing the nervous system") to the impressively technical ("contains the active ingredient hypericin, which acts as a monoamine oxidase inhibitor") to the openly defiant ("A new study shows the herb St. John's Wort might be just as effective as antidepressant drugs, and with fewer side effects").

Manufacturers can do this because they present the claims within the context of "information," providing some sketchy facts about the herb in general and quoting all too briefly from the summaries of a few studies without describing their limitations. Other companies edge around the rules by making overt medicinal claims, but follow up by placing a tiny disclaimer notice on their ads or packaging: "This information has not been evaluated by the Food and Drug Administration. This product is not intended to diagnose, treat, cure, or prevent any disease." Even if you're one of the few who do scrutinize fine print, the distinction between the claims and the cautionary statements that follow may be too subtle to make any real impression.

I've heard St. John's Wort described as an oil, a tincture (whatever that is), and a tea. Which should I use?

You see different preparations to treat different ailments. Basically, they divide into two categories: those preparations taken internally and those applied externally. Look at the chart on page 246 to see which preparations are indicated for a specific use (but see Chapter 7 for information on the limited proofs documented for many of these uses). For the record, tinctures are alcohol-based extracts—preparations where the herb has been left to soak in an alcohol base over a period of time to extract and preserve its potent oils.

I buy St. John's Wort tea. But the box doesn't say what's in it, let alone give levels of active ingredients. Am I getting enough hypericin?

The only one who can answer that question is the manufacturer—who is clearly not telling. And this is not at all uncommon, especially with herbal teas. One brand of St. John's Wort tea I found in a health-food store dedicated a lot of packaging space to its commitment to environmental responsibility and dedication to quality, but offered no ingredient listing, dosing information or even an address to write to with any questions or concerns. It clearly did not feel so dedicated to its consumers. You *could* track down a manufacturer's phone number and request independent documentation of its tea's active ingredients, plus a complete list of other ingredients. Instead, I'd simply shop around for a company that cares enough about their consumers to inform them of these basic facts and preferably offers a satisfaction guarantee. They are out there. Many brands provide dosage information as well, generally based on the "3 × 300 mg" model. (See more about dosing in Chapter 5.) I have noted teas ranging from 300 to around 900 milligrams of St. John's Wort per bag. Be cautious, though, in believing everything you read on these labels.

I'm taking capsules and feel a little dizzy. I don't know if it's the herb or not. Why don't packages list possible side effects?

For the same reason they are supposed to refrain from making therapeutic claims—because herbal therapies are not technically considered medicines in the U.S., just nutritional supplements. And the regulatory philosophy is that if it's not a medicine, it can't have "side effects." Still, I have noticed a few packages out there, notably Nature's Harvest products, which do post warnings about use in pregnant or lactating women, children, people consuming alcohol, and patients undergoing treatment for certain conditions. They also noted potential side effects to watch for. This is the exception, though, not the rule. Don't rely on packages to provide you with this information—or to tell you what to do if you experience any odd symptoms. Instead, if you notice any mental or physical side effects while on an herbal remedy or any other treatment, inform your doctor. (See Chapter Six for more about potential side effects relating to use of St. John's Wort.)

What does St. John's Wort taste like?

When in capsule form, it tastes like . . . well, a capsule. As an extract, its flavor is concentrated and can be bitter, but most people mix the extract into some applesauce or juice to mask any unpleasant taste. In prepackaged teas, the flavor is often barely discernible—St. John's Wort on its own makes a very weak and mild tea, something like a watered-down version of generic brand-name teas. However, some companies blend St. John's Wort with other ingredients that have stronger flavors, like fennel, cinnamon, spearmint, ginger, cardamom, cloves, or pepper. This produces nicely aromatic and occasionally spicy teas. Brewing tea from St. John's Wort you've dried yourself will yield a stronger cup of the pure herb, sometimes described as medicinal-tasting, but it is still a flavor easily overwhelmed or enhanced by other flavors, like licorice. Many people recommend honey or brown sugar for sweetening and deepening the taste. Other people have been known to take St. John's Wort in homemade alcohol-based concoctions like vinegars—even brandies and wines. Those will, of course, vary in taste owing the other flavorings added and the strength of

Form	How Taken	For
Cold infusions (teas, tisanes)	Internally or externally	A wide range of conditions and disorders ranging from depression (still being studied) to bronchitis, nausea, digestive problems, etc. (anecdotal) Externally mixed with water for washes (see below; anecdotal)
Alcohol-based extracts (tinctures, macerations)	Internally or externally	A wide range of conditions and disorders ranging from depression (still being studied) to bronchitis, bed-wetting, worms, nausea, digestive problems, etc. (anecdotal) Externally mixed with water for washes, see below (largely anecdotal)
Glycerin-based extracts	Internally	A wide range of conditions and disorders ranging from depression (still being studied) to bronchitis, bed-wetting, worms, nausea, digestive problems, etc. (anecdotal)
Infused oils	Internally or externally	Stomach upset in small doses (anecdotal) Externally: wounds, burns, sprains, or bruises, a massage oil for sore muscles (largely anecdotal)
Essential oils	Externally ONLY	Aromatherapy
Ointments (creams)	Externally	Wounds, burns, sprains, or bruises (largely anecdotal)

Form	How Taken	For
Capsules, pills, tablets	Internally	A wide range of conditions and disorders ranging from depression (still being studied) to digestive problems, etc. (anecdotal)
Washes (baths)	Externally	Wounds, burns, sprains, sore muscles, or bruises, from extract, tea or oil base (anecdotal)

the alcohol base. The therapeutic qualities of vinegars and wines remain untested for St. John's Wort.

When I make tea using a commercial brand it isn't red, like the oil from St. John's Wort. What color should it be?

Homemade teas produced by the pure dried herb are always reddish in hue. But commercial teas vary in color from a deep rusty wine to a pale gold, even after lengthy steeping. Some of those labeled with the greatest amounts of St. John's Wort were the lightest in color. Of course, the manufacturers may not be accurately reporting the amounts of the herb, and none of the commercial teas I've found so far has standardized ingredients. But more likely, the color was influenced by other ingredients added to the blend for flavor. If you're concerned about the content of your favorite brand, write or call the company that makes it and ask for documented information on its product. Or better yet, ask yourself. How do *you* feel on the treatment? If your doctor has approved it as part of your therapy and it's working, then don't worry about the color. If you're still uncertain, try a standardized extract or capsule, which would be more potent than teas in any case.

I heard that the ingredient that treats depression is stronger in capsule than tea form. Is that true?

It certainly looks that way. Both forms use the dried herb as their base, and some of the herb's oil is already lost in the drying process, but the water used in tea infusions further dilutes its potency. Plus, many of the capsules sold have reportedly been "standardized," to ensure more precise levels of active ingredients—none of the teas makes such a claim, and so they may have only trace amounts of the herb or its active constituents. The most potent way to take this herbal remedy is a liquid extract. Extracts, also called tinctures, are often sold in small, dark bottles with miniature eyedropper dispensers attached. Active ingredients work more effectively in extracts than the dried herb. The alcohol base used in most herbal extracts reacts chemically with the active ingredients and also helps preserve them. These extracts, or capsules which contain them, are the form of St. John's Wort most often tested on depression. Capsules are generally easier to find in the U.S. than liquid extracts—and many Americans are more comfortable taking this familiar-looking and convenient form of medicine—so look for those capsules which state they use standardized extracts as their base. A capsule form of St. John's Wort is being used in the study currently being performed by the National Institutes of Health (NIH).

Should I buy St. John's Wort oil? Is that the same as an extract?

No, oils are not the same as extracts. Both are made by soaking the herb, but extracts use a base of alcohol or glycerin, while oils use vegetable-oil bases. St. John's Wort oils have been used as a balm on cuts, bruises, and sprains, and there are a few anecdotal accounts that they could be effective on stomach upset in small doses, but these uses have not been the subject of definitive testing and nothing has been reported on the oil's use for treatment of depression. Stick to extracts for the purposes of depression therapy. If you do buy the oil for its other purposes, use caution—be sure you're not buying a product intended for aromatherapy. Aromatherapy oils are highly concentrated, far more so than medicinal extracts, and are sometimes called "essential oils." They are *never* intended to be taken internally for any reason or condition. Herbs that are beneficial in other forms can become highly poisonous to your system when ingested in this concentrated manner. To date, I have not seen St. John's Wort sold for aromatherapy, but its increased popularity and labeling as an "aromatic" might lead to its appearance in some aromatherapy lines. Many other herbs are currently available in both aromatherapy oils as well as medicinal oils intended to be taken internally, so confusion can occur. One man in Washington recently suffered kidney failure when he consumed an aromatherapy oil form of wormwood, mistaking it for absinthe, a liquor with wormwood as an ingredient. This potentially deadly misidentification is easy to avoid. As with any medication, check the label to be sure that it isn't toxic if swallowed. On the flip side, some oils labeled as "flower essences" are the basis for homeopathic remedies. These remedies are distilled until there is virtually no trace of the original herb present. This is considered by homeopaths as the proper way to dose with herbs, but no tests have been done using St. John's Wort in this manner. There is every indication that using the herb in this highly diluted form would be a waste of time, effort, and money. So, be careful when purchasing oils as balms, to be sure you're getting one safe for internal use or application to skin, and one that has the correct amount of the herb you need.

How come labels on capsules say they contain the "extract"? I thought an extract was a liquid?

Liquid extracts, as has been mentioned, are the liquids strained off after an herb has been left to soak in a mixture of grain alcohol and water for some weeks. But these fluid extracts can be further processed to remove all the liquids, leaving behind a solid material that is ground into powder to fill capsules. Even though dry extracts are made directly from liquid extracts, the liquid form is still considered more potent, because some of the volatile oils are lost in the additional processing.

After all the interest, I thought I'd be seeing St. John's Wort popping up all over the supplement shelves in stores. It's still hard for me to find.

That may be due to overexposure—some people report their local stores are sold out of St. John's Wort as a result of the recent media spotlight on the herb. Or, it may be the result of the past *under*exposure of St. John's Wort. The television reports that started all the recent hoopla are still just that—recent—and have only just begun to build a wave of public awareness. So you may not see St. John's Wort flood the big department chains or groceries near you until more manufacturers scramble to get on the bandwagon. Then, too, many stores fell victim to other herbal "fads" in the past and might be waiting to see if St. John's Wort is more than just hype. But given the herb's rising popularity, it seems certain you'll be seeing more products featuring St. John's Wort very soon, as stores either restock or more manufacturers respond to the increasing requests for this medicinal herb. In the meantime, your best bets are local health-food stores and specialty chains like General Nutrition Centers. If local stores don't stock it, ask them to place a special order for you. Or try contacting a manufacturer directly; some companies are listed in the resource chapter. And if you have access to the Internet, there's a whole spectrum of manufacturers and growers on-line just waiting to take your order. Many of these maintain web sites that provide informational content on the herb. The most responsible of these present the herb's colorful folklore and historical background as just that, and note that clinical proof of St. John's Wort's effectiveness does not yet exist. Others, though, boldly claim a variety of treatment uses, presenting these statements as if they were universally accepted and proven fact. They do this in a very convincing and impressive style. Be wary of some of these informational "sells," or you'll be persuaded into thinking St. John's Wort is a miracle cure before you have a chance to realize that these on-line distributors have no more claim to authority than the teenage clerk at your local New-Age shop. Often these web sites give an appearance of authenticity that can persuade you that *everything* they say is true. *Caveat emptor*—let the buyer beware!

Will the demand cause an increase in price?

Some St. John's Wort users have already noticed a jump in price for the herb, although the increases so far have not been substantial. It's hard to say how the industry will respond if the demand grows. Luckily, St. John's Wort is still so common a resource it remains very reasonably priced. Its easy availability may also help ensure higher levels of overall quality in its commercial preparation, because the more rare and expensive an herbal ingredient the more likely a company is to dilute it in its products by adding cheaper fillers to the mix. This is especially true in powder-based preparations like tablets, capsules and teas.

Is there any chance of St. John's Wort becoming endangered by overharvesting and getting harder to find?

That's a danger facing any popular product. Some manufacturers are already talking about the difficulty in finding quantities of the herb that produce the optimum potencies of hypericin. Whether this is a truthful assessment of the competition facing harvesters of the plant, or just a clever excuse for a possible rise in price is still unclear. As more people harvest their own St. John's Wort and more companies wildcraft existing crops rather than cultivate their own, it's certain some depletion will occur. Certainly the plant is ubiquitous now, but anyone who recalls the fate of the buffalo knows that a plentiful resource can become scarce quickly.

Where can I buy this stuff? Is it only available in health-food stores?

No, St. John's Wort is becoming available in just about every outlet that stocks vitamins, from organic health-food stores to groceries and conventional pharmacies to Wal-Marts. However, some forms, like bulk herbs, can still only be found in the smaller specialty shops. If you're having trouble finding the herb, make some phone calls. Look in your local phone book under the categories of "Herbs," "Health & Diet Food Products," and "Pharmacies." Under the latter two headings, start with those places that mention "botanicals" in their ads.

My health-food store doesn't stock any of the brands I've heard about. How can I choose the best brand-name tea or capsule from its selection?

Ask around. Your doctor and any specialists you visit should be the first you tap. See if they know of any brand that has a good reputation and which accurately reports St. John's Wort and hypericin content. If your physicians can't guide you, grill the salespeople at the local health-food stores. Ask at different stores to get a more balanced picture. See if they've had complaints or raves about any particular brand. Making it clear you'll be a repeat customer if it works may encourage them to share the facts rather than recommend the brand with the best short-term profit margin. Ask friends if they're taking it or know someone who is, and get recommendations. You might be surprised at how many of your acquaintances have tried St. John's Wort and are eager to share their discovery with others. If there's no one in your medical or social circle to consult, there are other options: Try contacting one of the herb and alternative-medicine organizations listed in the resource chapter. Check with your local Better Business Bureau to see if anyone has lodged a complaint against a particular brand (or even a local health-food store). Even with the recommendations from others, a particular brand may not be the best choice for you. There may be another more effective with your unique body chemistry. If you're experiencing no side effects, but haven't seen results after six weeks at recommended doses, switch to a different brand.

Can I use the Internet to find a good brand of St. John's Wort?

If you have access to the Internet or an on-line service, visit herbal or alternative-medicine chat rooms and message boards to see which brands other people with your condition are talking about. Target those sites dedicated to your particular illness or ailment. Be warned, though, that some "visitors" to these sites may be representatives from the very companies that sell St. John's Wort preparations. Ask questions to get a better picture of the person from whom you're taking advice. Bear in mind that some informational or newsgroup sites are sponsored by or linked to pages owned by herbal manufacturers. They might present a more rosy picture of the herb and their particular brand than is strictly true. Maintain a healthy skepticism when approaching information presented by people you don't know and whose credentials are difficult to check—good advice both on the web and in more virtual reality.

What are some of the reputable brand names out there? Name names!

Because they are the only ones tested extensively so far, I recommend the extracts manufactured in Germany, which are imported and repackaged by some American distributors. Some *Hypericum* buyers clubs exist. These are organized groups of users, usually comprised of AIDS sufferers or people combating that disease. They are reputable sources of these imported St. John's Wort remedies, although some people have reported problems with the prompt filling of orders, especially orders placed via the Internet. The following are standardized brands sold in Germany:

Hyperforat
Psychotonin M
Jarsin
Neuroplant
Sedariston

In the United States, they are more often found under different names. One of the most common is a brand called Kira, distributed by Lichtwer Pharmaceuticals in the U.S. in tablet form. Kira uses an extract, LI-160, which was utilized in many of the clinical trials conducted in Germany.

I heard St. John's Wort products contain alcohol. What can I do if I have to avoid alcohol?

Most liquid extracts of St. John's Wort use alcohol as their base. However, some brands take additional steps to remove the alcohol after the extract is made. It involves a simple process that utilizes evaporation. These brands generally substitute glycerin for the alcohol as a preservative. Other brands use glycerin from the beginning. And, of course, there are the options of capsules or teas, which although less potent are still valid choices. Certainly, anyone who would be at risk using alcohol-based products should read labels very carefully and select from the many options which don't contain alcohol as an ingredient. But remember, there's still debate over whether so-called "special populations"—children, pregnant or lactating women, or people with addiction problems—should be using herbal remedies at all.

If quality levels vary from brand to brand and even box to box, how can I ensure a consistent dose each time?

Although levels may vary from bottle to bottle, they will still remain more consistent within the same brand than if your purchases shift between different manufacturers. So try to use the same brand throughout your course of treatment, unless it is simply not working. Then you'd want to experiment with another, as long as your doctor sees no reason to discontinue use of St. John's Wort. Choosing "standardized," one-ingredient herbal extracts, tablets, or capsules will help ensure the best possible consistency within a brand.

I can't swallow pills or capsules. What form of St. John's Wort should I buy?

Look for liquid extracts of St. John's Wort, usually sold in small, amber-colored glass bottles with eyedroppers attached. These extracts are more potent than capsules in any case, and can be taken mixed in juice, applesauce, honey, or teas. Check to be sure the herb has been standardized for its hypericin content. If you are unable to locate this form of the herb, you could try breaking open a capsule into juice or applesauce and taking the powdered herb that way. Be warned, however, that this approach is not recommended for some medications—often the capsule helps control the time-release nature of active ingredients or protects your mouth and throat.

Which of the brands of the herbal version of Phen-Fen is the best?

That's easy: None. There are increasing numbers of herb-based answers to the Phen-Fen backlash appearing on supplement shelves. These are being sold under names that more than suggest the Phen-Fen connection, like Herbal Phen Fuel, DietPhen, or No-Phen. St. John's Wort is cropping up as an ingredient in some of these mixtures, not so much because it targets appetite as for its apparent effects on the depression that's sometimes the culprit behind overeating. There's very little evidence to suggest these herbal Phen-Fens work—even anecdotal support is slight and usually mixed. However, the biggest argument against buying any of these products is the fact that these mixtures often combine St. John's Wort with *Ephedra*. The FDA is currently investigating complaints about strong reactions to mixtures containing *Ephedra*, also known as Ma Huang. So steer clear of any products making claims about weight loss or those that contain St. John's Wort in combination with other herbs that may not be as safe.

My favorite brand of St. John's Wort says it's been "wildcrafted." What does *that* mean?

When a product has been "wildcrafted," that means it's been made using plants that were harvested in the wild, rather than gathered from cultivated plants. This doesn't necessarily mean that the manufacturer's employees are roaming through forests looking for the odd St. John's Wort plant. The company may own whole meadows containing virtually nothing but St. John's Wort. But a certain amount of control has been surrendered and the plant is allowed to grow at its own pace— it is never forced as cultivated plants sometimes are. People who harvest St. John's Wort on their own, using plants that have not been cultivated, are called wildcrafters.

How much should I take?

When buying commercial preparations, you should follow the recommended doses given on the package. If a range of doses are indicated, start with the lowest one listed, to gauge side effects and test the herb's effectiveness. Obviously, if the low dose works, you wouldn't want to take more than was needed. And if the low dose produces unpleasant side effects, you wouldn't want to experiment with even greater amounts. (See Chapter 5 for more information about the doses that are used to treat depression.)

If I can't rely on the truthful labeling or consistency of commercial St. John's Wort products, can't I just grow it myself?

You might be growing it already; check your backyard. St. John's Wort is so common in some North American regions that it is vilified as a "pest" plant or weed. Ranchers wage an all-out war against the stuff, which grows freely over their cattle ranges but does not interact as well with livestock as it appears to with humans. (See more about St. John's Wort's effects on cattle in Chapter 4.) The plant is hardy in most American zones, and seems to do especially well in poor soil—popping up like a determined jack-in-the-box wherever you find deforested areas, overgrazed pastures, or other patches of disturbed earth. Many people use various species of St. John's Wort as attractive borders and ground covers, even the *Hypericum perforatum* species used in the treatment of depression. Its flowers are attractive enough to make it a decorative as well as medicinal plant. But remember, the decision to use homegrown medicinals is one not taken lightly.

Confer with medical professionals and herbal experts before taking that step, and read through the general guidelines and cautions for growing and harvesting St. John's Wort in the following chapter.

EIGHT

✎

Homegrown Remedies: The Basics on Harvesting and Preparing Your Own St. John's Wort

Jen suffered from bouts of winter depression almost every year. Her doctor had known for some time that Jen was using St. John's Wort tablets to augment her phototherapy. No side effects had arisen from her use of the herb except for a few days of mild stomach upset. Jen felt St. John's Wort helped keep her emotions on an even keel, especially on days when she could not make time for a light therapy session. But one day, Jen dropped something of a bombshell during a session; she casually told her doctor that the St. John's Wort no longer seemed to be working as well. "Maybe," she said, "it's because I've been using St. John's Wort my friend picked and dried herself, instead of the stuff I've been buying at the store." Jen's doctor asked her to tell him more about her friend's methods for picking and preparing the homegrown remedy. "It grows everywhere," Jen shrugged. Her friend had learned to dry flowers for crafts and had prepared a batch of St. John's Wort from plants she had found growing wild in the fields. All of this did not sound good to Jen's doctor, who told her that she might be seeing a difference in the way the herb worked for a number of reasons. Perhaps the crops her friend picked from did not have a high concentration of the oils and other ingredients needed to fight mood disorder. The plants might not have been picked at the correct time or dried in a way that preserved their active contents. It was possible her friend was not picking St. John's Wort at all, but some similar-looking flower. Worse, the plants could have been exposed to airborne toxins if they had not been protected from weed and pest-control sprays. Jen's doctor suggested that she toss the rest of her friend's mixture in the trash and return to her old dose of standardized tablets. A month later, Jen was back. She was starting to notice "a big difference" after just three weeks on standardized St. John's Wort, and had advised her friend to stick to making wreaths.

In today's arena of competitive sound bites and Internet chat rooms, there's been an incredible surge in the flow of information—and misinformation—about every conceivable subject under the sun. As a result of their high potential for human drama and the intense interest they inspire, medical breakthroughs seem to head the list.

St. John's Wort is a perfect case in point. The recent media attention has created a groundswell of information, both true, false, and the gray area of "not proven" that falls somewhere in between. Since the individuals who actively search out information about treating their conditions are often the more independent among us, and the ones open to alternative treatments like St. John's Wort perhaps more independent still, it's no surprise that many of these same people decide to take full control over their use of this new therapy. They quickly move beyond the questions of "Is St. John's Wort an option for me?" and "Where do I buy it?" to "Why can't I grow and make this on my own?"

That's one of the places where the rapid exchange of information can be dangerous as well as helpful. Depression sufferers see TV reports and pause to pick St. John's Wort from the roadside on their way home. Others, hearing about the new popularity of the herb, stop spraying their backyard crops with weed killer and begin harvesting it instead. Some swap dubious hints for home remedies, using recipes they've gotten from "a friend who knows someone who grows it."

As a psychiatrist, herbal gardening advice is not exactly my strong suit. But concern over the improper ways people are collecting and dishing up doses of homegrown St. John's Wort has motivated this chapter. In it, you'll find cautions for harvesters of both wildcrafted and cultivated herbs and some basic guidelines for more careful collecting. You'll find a chart giving equivalents for measurements commonly used in homegrown remedies. These may help you avoid confusion since many Americans are unfamiliar with the metric-based amounts given in some traditional herbals. There are a few basic "recipes" for remedies, as well—more to steer you away from others you may run across that are way off base than to give you a detailed step-by-step process for making them at home.

These guidelines have been harvested from some of the most recent, reputable herbal references as well as the most definitive traditional sources. Still, these guidelines are no substitute for genuine hands-on know-how. If you are determined to try your hand at making St. John's Wort remedies, do so responsibly and intelligently: make them under the watchful eye of an experienced herbalist the first time you try them. You'll find some ideas for locating these experts in the resource chapter.

Remember, the preparations described later in this chapter are predicated on your collecting the correct plants in the first place, and getting a healthy harvest. And—this can't be stressed enough—you can never be sure what kind of potency you're achieving in homemade remedies. If ensuring an accurate dosage—one that's been clinically tested for the treatment of depression—is important to you, it's better to purchase commercial brands in standardized doses from a source you trust.

Some people will never progress beyond the belief that natural medicines are best for whatever ails you. Certainly, "natural" is good, but science and technology are not the enemy in treating depression or any other disorder—think about that the next time you pull a traditional homegrown remedy off the World Wide Web.

If this stuff grows everywhere, why bother to buy it?

That's exactly what pharmaceutical companies are afraid you'll say about St. John's Wort and other herb products. The

fact that St. John's Wort grows like a weed across much of
the U.S. is one reason pharmaceutical companies here are reluctant to invest in research into its effectiveness. If it grows
by the side of the road, free for anyone to pick, they reason,
why spend millions in testing it? These companies see no incentive for investing money in a medication for which they
may see no return. Of course, in Germany manufacturers profit
from sales of the herb even though it's widely available in
over-the-counter preparations and can be grown there as well.
People in that country purchase the prescription "drug" form
of the herb because they know the pharmaceutical grade St.
John's Wort contains regulated, standardized doses. Besides,
the purchase of St. John's Wort with a prescription can be
reimbursed by health insurance. Here in the U.S., the best
reason to buy is because reputable manufacturers test their
products to ensure the standard levels of hypericin, something
you can't achieve at home.

I've decided to plant a medicinal herb garden. Is there anything I should know about cultivating my own St. John's Wort?

Cultivating St. John's Wort is fairly simple, since it has the
hardiness of a weed. You can start St. John's Wort from a
seed or by root propagation. Speciality seed companies or
nurseries with large herbal sections may carry the seeds or,
less frequently, young plants. St. John's Wort's seeds are tiny;
a goodly number of them are crammed into each of the
flower's three-celled seed capsules. Break open the pod when
you're ready to plant, but first the seeds must be germinated.
Briefly, germination requires that you freeze the seeds until
it's time to plant (or that they are started in ground that will
remain frozen for some weeks). Find out more about ensuring
your germination is successful from your seed provider. If you
harvest your own seeds, be sure to reserve some for reseeding
the area you collected from, or allow some seeds to fall before
you begin your seed hunt.

Once established, St. John's Wort spreads easily and can
occasionally overwhelm a garden. Plant it in sun or light shade
(although it appears to be more potent when grown in full
sun). This herb is a perennial, so it will return after a killing
winter, and seems to do well when you just leave it alone.

Some herbalists feel that the plant becomes more potent if it's not coddled, and it certainly thrives in spots where other plants fail. It does grow best when the soil has good drainage, however. Too much care often results in overwatering, so most gardeners and herbalists offer the advice that you plant it, then ignore it until it's ready for harvesting. They also recommend waiting until the second year to begin harvesting, as the potency of this particular herb seems enhanced as the plant matures.

However, the most important rule for cultivating St. John's Wort, if you're growing it for therapeutic use, is never to use any but organic pest control on your St. John's Wort or anywhere else in your garden. Pesticides and weed killers can reach the plant through the soil even if you're not using them in the same plot as your herb, unless your St. John's Wort is planted in a nonporous container. Even then, airborne chemicals can contaminate your herb.

Any words of warning for the amateur herb gardener?

First, make sure your seeds or starter plants were accurately identified as St. John's Wort in the first place. Be sure to confirm the plant's ID when it is in full bloom. There are a lot of members of the *Hypericum* family, and even expert herbalists sometimes make mistakes when harvesting a plant.

Another note of caution: Just because it's common and easy to grow doesn't mean you should wildcraft or cultivate your own St. John's Wort—getting the right levels of active ingredients is at best a crapshoot with homemade remedies and especially problematical in the case of an herb like St. John's Wort, where the identity and interplay of active ingredients is largely unknown. Don't forget that no one is really sure which of the complex constituents in St. John's Wort is responsible for its apparent therapeutic effects. Even if you were using the 0.3% hypericin level as your gauge, there's no way you'll know exactly what concentration is in any given plant you grow unless you happen to have a chromatography device in your home! It's proven difficult to control these levels even in professionally cultivated plants grown under uniform conditions.

Finally, inexperienced gardeners can make mistakes that will lessen the herb's effectiveness at best, or cause toxic reactions in a worst-case scenario. Unless you're an expert, don't go it alone. And if you're seriously unwell, seek medical help and guidance to find a more effective therapy for your disorder.

I'm ready to run out and pick St. John's Wort myself. What does it look like?

The first rule of herbalism: Make sure you've correctly identified the plant you want to pick. See Chapter One for a description of St. John's Wort, and refer to the following drawing. But neither of these is really enough to be your guide, since many wildflowers look alike, and there are so many species even within the *Hypericum* family. In the 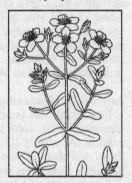 best of all worlds, you'd ask the advice of a botanical society or experienced herbalist before harvesting St. John's Wort yourself. If they can't come to you, go to them. Take a photograph of the plant you *think* is St. John's Wort in its natural setting. Bring your photo, along with an uncrushed clipping, to an expert willing to give you a few minutes of his or her time. Or, sign up for a botanical hike; they're offered in many communities. Choose one in late June or early July, so you'll know exactly what the herb looks like at the time when you'd normally harvest it. Let the guide know of your interest in identifying St. John's Wort. As a last resort, purchase an herb book with good, clear photos of the herb—some are suggested in the resource chapter. Bring one of them with you on your harvest, to be sure you're getting what you intend to, and cross-check it with others when you return home.

Can I pick any species of St. John's Wort?

If you're picking St. John's Wort for the purpose of treating depression, then no, not all species in the family are created equal. Be sure you're harvesting *Hypericum perforatum* and not one of its relatives like *H. calycinum*, also known as Aaron's-Beard. *Calycinum* is a lush, lower-growing member of the family that is sometimes planted as ground cover. Even though other *Hypericum* relatives, like *H. hirsutum* and *H.*

puctatum also contain hypericin and other active constituents, they have not been tested for treatment of depression and the concentrations of the constituents may not produce the same effects.

My friend showed me some St. John's Wort growing by the side of the road and said I can find it anywhere. Is it all right to pick if it's growing like a weed?

It's true that St. John's Wort can be found growing wild in meadows and forests, as well as empty lots, roadsides, and slag heaps in many parts of North America. However, you would never want to pick some of these plants, because of their possible exposure to toxic contaminants. Some people do brag that they pick St. John's Wort from alongside the road on their way home each day. That's not wise. As your mother would say: You don't know where it's been. Or rather, you don't know what it's been in contact with. For that reason, you should not harvest plants that grow along popular well-traveled animal trails, where they're more likely to have been exposed to natural contaminants such as dog urine, or from areas that might have been sprayed with pesticides. That means avoiding any plant "by the side of the road." Plants have been known to absorb up to twenty times their natural levels of lead from car exhaust—yet another reason not to pick plants less than a mile from major roadways. Washing the herb isn't the answer in these situations, either. It may not remove the contaminants, and even gentle handling may break open oil glands in the leaves.

What other tips should I keep in mind when picking wild or cultivated St. John's Wort?

There are a number of guidelines that anyone should keep in mind when harvesting medicinal plants, and some that are particular to St. John's Wort:

When should I harvest?

You should avoid picking herbs that are damp from dew or rain—moisture promotes the growth of mold. So wait for a dry day, one sunny enough to burn off the morning's condensation. Pick as early in the day as possible after the dew has dried.

St. John's Wort is considered by many herbalists to be at
its most potent right before and during flowering. Fortunately,
it's easy to schedule a harvesting date because the plant generally blossoms at a very specific time of year—on or near
June 24, St. John's Day, which accounts for the plant's common name. In the United States, St. John's Wort blooms
through August. Some people report that if they make a harvest in early July, they'll get a second flowering and another
harvest late in August or early September.

Which plants should I pick from?
First, be sure you're picking from a stand of the correct species
of St. John's Wort, *Hypericum perforatum*. Get the most positive ID possible. Bring a sample of the flowering plant to a
local nursery, herbalist, or botanical society to get an expert
opinion. On the day of your harvest, take one or more detailed
plant guides with you (see resource chapter for some recommendations), for a final check.

Once you're sure what you've got really is a crop of St.
John's Wort, be selective. Choose the plants you harvest carefully, clipping only from those that are the most healthy. How
can you tell? Healthy plants will have whole, upright leaves
and blooms, both showing strong colors. Pass over those
plants with dark spots or patches on their leaves and stems.
Avoid clipping from plants that seem lifeless and limp. Pick
flowers that still have most of their five petals. Harvest from
large "stands," or crops, of the herb. Their greater numbers
will more easily support the loss of a few plants. Don't choose
plants closer than one mile to major roads or any that might
have been sprayed with weed killer or pesticide, such as plants
found in vacant lots or along roadsides. One good place to
look is alongside the borders of organic farms, as those areas
are less likely to be contaminated by toxic pest and weed controls. But be sure you're not harvesting in places you wouldn't
be welcome. Ask around: Is the land owned by someone who
would not appreciate amateur herbalists popping up while he's
mowing the lawn? Are the plants in that area protected for
some reason? Could you be damaging a fragile environment
if you harvest from that location? Check to be sure you don't
need permission to pick plants from any site.

How should I pick it?

Think long-term when harvesting St. John's Wort: Leave enough of the plant so it will be able to return the following year. Don't yank the plant up by its roots or cut the herb back by more than a half. You won't need the root in any case, except if you want to propagate the plant elsewhere, like your garden. In that case you'd use care to get the root intact. Therapeutic preparations of St. John's Wort utilize only the ariel parts of the plant; not surprisingly that means those parts exposed to the air, such as the flowers, stems, leaves, and seed capsules. In addition, this herb appears to be most potent in the topmost portions of the plant. You are best off harvesting only the top two inches of each flowering stem, leaving a few on here and there, along with their seed capsules, to enable the crop to reseed itself. St. John's Wort's leaves contain pockets of a volatile red oil. When popped open, this oil can stain your fingers, and some herbalists have reported getting rashes when harvesting the plant with bare hands. Wearing gardening gloves when harvesting seems a sensible precaution, especially if you have sensitive skin.

Then what?

Depopulate your plants. Pick through them in the field and back at home, remembering to check inside the buds and under the leaves for bugs and foreign matter like cobwebs. When transporting the herb from the wild to your home, try to avoid crushing it. Any damage to the leaves and flowers will release the potent volatile oils. Carry your clippings gingerly in a paper bag. Label the bag with St. John's Wort's Latin name before you leave home, and do the same on any more permanent storage containers for the herb. Label every preparation you make with the Latin name for clarity of identification, the common name St. John's Wort for instant recognition, the dates the herb was harvested and prepared, the parts of the herb used, location found, and any other ingredients in the mix. These are all facts that later will help you make the most consistent batches possible, target problems if you have adverse reactions to any preparation, and alert you to which batches may be past their potency.

I grow St. John's Wort in my garden and pick the fresh herbs in summer to use for tea. But I only get the blues in the middle of winter—like clockwork. What then?

It sounds like you should speak with your physician about SAD, seasonal affective disorder. If together you decide St. John's Wort is a sound treatment option, and that it's a good idea to continue harvesting your own, you might try drying the herb for later use or storing extracts you make from the fresh leaves. Read on in this chapter for some recommendations and cautions about producing these homemade remedies. Of course, you could simply augment your homegrown therapies with commercial brands during the rest of the year. I would recommend liquid extracts or capsules for this purpose, rather than commercially sold teas, because teas are rarely, if ever, standardized for active ingredients. They may be far less potent than your own home brews. For those who rely on commercial sources for the herb, and are concerned that even some commercial brands rely on wildcrafting, the good news is that St. John's Wort also grows in Australia. It flourishes there during our own winter season, so can be harvested in the wild virtually year-round.

I want to keep a supply of the dried herb on hand to use in different ways all year. How do I dry St. John's Wort?

It's best to use the fresh herb to make liquid extractions with an alcohol base. It's the most potent form of herbal preparation and can be stored for up to a year, long enough to wait out the next harvest. But if liquid extracts aren't an option, the first step in the preparation of your herb is drying it. St. John's Wort contains volatile oils, which do not respond as well to the quicker method of oven drying; that means air-drying it. Air-drying is not a speedy process—it can take anywhere from six days to six weeks, although every day that goes by may reduce the potency of your St. John's Wort. Find a place where the drying herb won't be exposed to full sunlight (since light during drying can affect potency) and where it will get little or no moisture. Choose a spot where the herbs will be out of the reach of small children. Arrange flowers or whole stems of St. John's Wort in single layers on fine mesh trays (clean new sections of screen doors or windows have been known to work well) or on plain trays lined with unbleached paper or parchment. The herbs should be bone-dry when beginning this process, or mold can contaminate the whole tray. Wipe any damp patches with a cloth until completely dry, or cut them off and dispose of them. Turn the herbs each day to ensure even drying. Another drying method is available if you have cut whole stems instead of just picking flowers. You can tie stems into bundles of no more than eight and hang them upside down to dry. Then follow the same guidelines given for tray-drying in regard to moisture and sun exposure. Don't dry your herbs in garages or other places where strong or noxious odors may be absorbed by the herb. Those oils pick up everything! Drying is complete when the leaves are brittle and stems snap easily, but before the herb becomes powdery. Crumble the herb parts together and store as described later in this chapter.

How do you make the various preparations called for in different treatments?

Note: The following preparations are best attempted the first time under the watchful eye of someone who's been there before: an herbalist or naturalist with some experience in preparing herbal remedies. (See Chapter Nine for guidance in finding someone to help.)

It seems clear the most potent form of St. John's Wort is the alcohol-based extract, also called a tincture. Extracts form the basis of the doses given to many of the patients in existing clinical trials abroad. However, for one reason or another, people are using other forms of the herb as well. The more popular preparations are described in the pages that follow. When dosages are given, keep in mind that you can never be sure just how much of an active ingredient is present in any homegrown or wildcrafted harvest. Always start on the low end to test your body's tolerances and because it's always best to use the lowest dose that works for you of any medication, be it herbal or synthetic. If nothing is happening, you can increase the dose in small increments, never exceeding the standard amounts. Let your doctor know that you've made these preparations yourself and exactly how you're taking them.

Materials:
For any of these herbal preparations, you must begin with clean, dry herbs. Gently brush excess dirt off the herbs with

a cloth—if you're not sure whether your plants have been protected from pesticides and weed killer, don't use them. (St. John's Wort is a frequent victim of the latter, since it grows like a weed and is actively targeted by ranchers with livestock.) Pick through your plants to remove foreign matter and bugs, checking inside each flower or bud and under the leaves. When making homegrown preparations, some ambitious amateur herbalists use only the flower heads, thinking these are the source of the herb's potency. This is not a good idea for two reasons: first, it's a very time-consuming task; even cutting larger portions of the herbs, complete with leaves and stem, can be a slow business when you're selecting only healthy specimens. Second, no one is sure exactly which are the active constituents in St. John's Wort; hypericin is just the best guess so far. Neither do we know exactly where in the plant these ingredients are in the most supply. In fact, the complex way the various elements interact within the whole plant may play a role in the therapeutic effects of the herb. Targeting just one part of this particular plant may be a mistake.

Utensils:
Several of the processes that follow involve heating water or some mixture containing the herbs; you should choose the cooking utensils needed carefully. Select a small heat-proof glass or enameled pan. Try to avoid using metal pans. These might add to the bitter taste of the herb, and aluminum or copper pans have the potential to release particles into your digestive system. Your measuring cups should ideally be heat-proof glass or polymer. Scales regularly tested for accuracy are a good idea, too, in order to weigh out the herbs. Most of these herbal preparations require a step where you're straining off the liquid from the rest of the plant. You can use a standard tea strainer for this, or substitute any fine mesh or gauze material.

Cold Infusions (aka. teas or tisanes):
When preparing infusions—what most of us would call teas—you should make only the amount needed that day. Cold infusions lose their potency fairly quickly since they are so diluted. Use these standard ratios of St. John's Wort to water:

1–2 teaspoons (about 2–3½ grams) dried St. John's
   Wort per cupful of water (start at the low end to
   check for tolerance)
OR
1 ounce dried St. John's Wort per pint of water
OR
3 teaspoons chopped fresh herb per cupful
OR
3 tablespoons chopped fresh herb per pint

Never boil water with the herb already in it. Such high
temperatures would result in steaming off the critical volatile
oils. Instead, you'll be pouring hot water over the herb and
then straining the infusion.

These instructions are for a day's supply of St. John's Wort
infusion, rather than a single cupful: Measure a pint of water
into a small pan. Do not begin with warm water; cold water
is best. Place over heat until water is just boiling. Remove
from heat and let stand about thirty seconds. This is called
taking the water "just off the boil" and will ensure that the
overheated liquid will not evaporate oils when you pour it over
the herb. When water has cooled for that half minute, spoon
in the herb or pour over herb in another glass, porcelain or
enameled container. Cover it if you have a lid and let steep
about ten minutes. You might gently stir the herb once or
twice during this time to release more oil. Place a strainer over
the mouth of the container you'll be using to store the infusion
(an airtight glass container is best). Pour the herb mixture
through the strainer into the container, so the plant material is
left in the strainer. For a stronger infusion, pour the liquid
through the plant material one more time. When you're
through straining, pour out a cupful (tea purists warm the cup
for each serving by swishing some warm water inside, before
adding the infusion). Store the remaining infusion in an airtight container in the refrigerator for another dose later in the
day. Two or three cupfuls are generally taken in a day. Depending on the potency of the infusion, start with one to two
cupfuls at first, to gauge your reaction. Drink the St. John's
Wort infusion hot or cold, sweetened with honey or brown
sugar, or flavored with licorice root. Some people who plan
on using the remedy over a long period save time by making

up homemade tea bags with premeasured amounts of the herb, which saves on straining too. You can find small muslin bags for this purpose in health food and some craft stores. Others freeze the strained liquid in concentrated quantities, using a ratio of 1 tablespoon of the herb to each cup of water. This concentrate is used to fill ice-cube trays; cubes are popped out and defrosted in warm water for tea.

Infused Oils:
Oils are most often used in external applications, as a balm for shallow cuts, for bruises, sprains, and minor burns. Very small doses taken internally have been used for stomach upset, but only in an anecdotal way.

To prepare oils, you'll need a glass jar with an airtight lid, of sufficient size to hold your harvest of St. John's Wort. Try working with something no larger than a pint at first; you might be surprised how many cuttings you'll need to fill it, as you'll be stuffing the jar with close-packed layers of the herb. If you're using just the flowers, first crush about four ounces in a tablespoon of vegetable oil. Almond, sunflower, and olive oil are most often recommended, although grapeseed, sesame oil, and plain vegetable oil are used as well. If you're processing whole stems, crush all parts together, using rubber gloves if your skin is sensitive to the volatile oils. Tightly pack the St. John's Wort into the jar. Then pour more of the vegetable-based oil inside, topping off the jar so the leaves are completely covered. Screw the lid on tightly. Find a spot that gets sun or indirect heat and leave the St. John's Wort to soak. After two to six weeks your oil is fully infused and should be a vibrant crimson, described by one herbalist as "cherry–Life Saver red." Start by soaking your St. John's Wort for only two weeks, trying longer periods only if the oil doesn't seem effective as a balm. Strain the oily mass through a fine mesh or cheesecloth into another clean jar. Leave it alone for 1 or 2 days to allow any moisture to collect at the bottom. You don't want this water in your stored oil. After it's separated, pour off the oil into an amber glass or glazed-earthenware storage container with airtight lid. Oils made this way will keep for up to a year if stored properly in a cool dry place.

Extracts (aka tinctures or macerations):

Extracts typically use an alcohol base diluted with water to make the most potent herbal preparation you can ingest. The water and alcohol break down different parts of the herb, so work very well in tandem. In addition, alcohol acts as a preservative, allowing for storage for up to a year. A strong note of caution, though: Use the correct type of alcohol! *Never* use wood alcohol, isopropyl rubbing alcohol, or alcohol labeled as methanol, methylated spirits, or methyl alcohol. These are highly toxic—even poisonous—if taken internally.

Commercial brands of St. John's Wort generally use ethyl alcohol tempered with water for the base of their extracts, but for home remedies diluted spirits of no less than 60 proof are often preferred. Vodka is usually the spirit of choice because of its purity: it has few additives.

Pour one pint of spirit into a glass container with an airtight lid. A jar with screw-on cap is fine; amber or another tinted glass is best. Add St. John's Wort to one pint of alcohol (½ liter). Eight ounces of the chopped fresh herb are called for, while only four ounces of dried herb are needed as there's less water content. Screw the lid on tightly. Now, store the jar someplace warm or sunny. Herbal references disagree on the length of time it needs to "ferment"—giving times ranging from two to eight weeks. Begin your extract experience with tinctures that have soaked for just two weeks. See how potent and effective these extracts are in your therapy before fermenting the herbs for longer periods. You should shake the jar at least once a day as it soaks. At the end of this period, strain the inert plant materials from the liquid using a fine mesh strainer or cheesecloth. Store your strained extract in the smallest container that will hold the extract. Measure the doses into a glass of water, hot or cold. To mask bitterness, you can add the extract to juice, a spoonful of honey, or a serving of applesauce instead of the water. When you buy commercial brands of extract, they often come in bottles stoppered with small eyedrop dispensers. A reputable manufacturer will have standardized the extract and produced droppers with fairly uniform apertures—the holes from which each drop falls. They are therefore able to recommend doses measured by drop, usually a range of 5–15 of them. Combine the uncertain potencies of homegrown remedies and the wide variety of droppers available (different size apertures can create a range of around 40–170 drops per fluid dram) and you create a high number of variables. Rather than use a dropper to measure doses, then, you might begin by using ½ teaspoon of the extract in 8 ounces of water each day. Work your way up to no more than 1½ teaspoons if the lower dose is not effective.

Extract Alternatives:

Options exist for those who are unable or unwilling to take alcohol but who want the strength of an alcohol-based tincture. When you're ready for your dose, measure out the correct amount of extract into a teacup or coffee mug. In a separate pan, heat a small amount of water to near-boiling point. (If the water boils, remove it from heat and let it sit for about fifteen seconds.) Then pour two tablespoons of the hot water over the tincture dose. Let the diluted extract stand for two minutes to allow the heat to evaporate most of the alcohol.

Glycerin is a syrupy-sweet substance available at pharmacies and some groceries; it can be used in place of alcohol in the production of extracts. This offers another alternative for the many people for whom even trace amounts of alcohol are unacceptable. Glycerin may not break down some of St. John's Wort's oils as well as alcohol, but it's still a better bet in terms of potency than a tea infusion. To make this type of infusion, you would use a ratio of one pint of glycerin plus one pint of water to every four ounces of dried St. John's Wort. If using fresh herbs, subtract ⅔ of the water from the ratio.

Apple-cider vinegar can replace the alcohol in another kind of tincture. It's suitable for use in cooking, but its therapeutic effects in the case of St. John's Wort are unknown.

Capsules:

Homemade capsules are produced by scooping dried and powdered herbs into empty gelatin capsules. Commercial capsules of St. John's Wort generally contain the standardized extract, mixed with inert fillers, to ensure the 0.3% hypericin level that seems optimum per dose. This is not a process you could duplicate with any accuracy in your home, so if you want to use capsules, I'd recommend purchasing standardized capsules from a reputable company, rather than making them yourself.

Ointments (aka salves or creams):

Ointments are applied to the skin for external applications on bruises, wounds, burns, and sprains. Remember that St. John's Wort's effectiveness for these uses has not been extensively studied or definitely proved; success in this use is largely anecdotal.

Some ointments simply form a protective layer; others become absorbed by the skin. To make a very basic ointment, place the harvested St. John's Wort into an enamel or heat-proof glass saucepan along with some Vaseline or petroleum jelly. Use the ratio of roughly four parts herb to one part jelly, i.e. 2 tablespoons of St. John's Wort to seven or eight ounces of the jelly. Warm the mixture gently. Do not allow it to boil, just to simmer. You want to liquefy the ingredients enough to blend them, not cook them. One way to control heating is by placing the jelly in a bowl inside the pan of water or by using a double boiler. Leave the mixture on this gentle heat for a period from fifteen minutes to an hour. If you're using fresh St. John's Wort instead of dried, it takes longer, because you have to be sure that all water from the plant has evaporated, or your ointment will spoil. When it's been heated long enough to blend the elements and steam off any moisture, pour the liquid through a strainer—clean gauze works well—into a clean glass heat-proof jar. Use caution, because the mixture will be hot. Don't seal the jar until the mixture has had a chance to cool, or you'll trap dampness inside. Store in a cool dark place; many people use their refrigerator.

Different bases will result in ointments that range from greasy oils to thick pastes. To make a creamier ointment, you might add some additional steps: After the petroleum jelly mixture has been strained, return it to the pan. Add a vegetable oil (such as olive oil) or fat (like lanolin or cocoa butter). Simmer to blend, and to remove any moisture. Stir in some beeswax to thicken the ointment and add a drop of benzoic tincture (available at pharmacies), for every ounce of fat-based ingredient used. That will help prevent the ointment from spoiling. Then, spoon into a wide-mouth jar or other clean container. When working with thicker, less-liquid ointments, try spreading a thick layer all along the sides and into every corner of the container before scooping the rest into the middle. That precaution will reduce the chance of any air pockets, which could promote quicker decay.

Washes (aka baths):
An herbal wash made from St. John's Wort is sometimes used to bathe sore feet or tennis elbows, to wash wounds, sores, or bruises. Remember, though, that the effectiveness of this use is largely anecdotal. A wash is simply a diluted form of any oil, tincture or infusion of an herb. Use any of the St. John's Wort preparations you've made as bases and add water. Use the wash to soak a sterile cotton pad or pour into a clean spray bottle. You can sometimes find glass spray bottles, but if forced to use plastic consider it a temporary housing, since St. John's Wort's volatile oils will interact with that material over time.

How should I store my St. John's Wort preparations once I've made them?

Correct storage is important with St. John's Wort, as with any herb, because you have already lost some of the herb's potent constituents in processing the plant. Improper storage will just leach more away every day, since air, light, heat, and age can eventually render even the most potent extract useless. Teas should be consumed the same day, so storage is less of an issue. Other preparations should be kept in glass, enameled metal or glazed-ceramic containers. Darker glass containers, such as amber-tinted varieties, are best. Keep your remedies in a cool, dry place. Some people store their St. John's Wort remedies in the refrigerator, but watch out for moisture if your container isn't really airtight. Label every container in which you store a medicinal herb—indicate Latin name, common name, date harvested, location of harvest, date prepared, and parts of the plant used. This information can prove invaluable in tracking problems with a batch or in pinpointing the combination of factors that produces the most effective preparation.

How should I store my dried St. John's Wort or other herbal preparations?

Although light and heat are needed to dry plants, and there is some indication that St. John's Wort responds favorably to light exposure in some situations, both these elements can lower an herb's potency over time. So, as soon as your herb has dried or you've finished making a therapeutic remedy, store it in a moisture-proof, light-barricading container. St. John's Wort contains volatile oils. Even after drying, these oils are present, and seem necessary to the herb's potency as a therapeutic. Plastic containers draw oils out of the herb, so it's best stored in dark glass, porcelain, or enameled-metal containers. Plain metals can impart a bitter taste to the herb. Oxygen is another element to avoid when storing herbs. Your containers should have airtight seals. Choose the smallest container needed to store your preparation and shift the contents to ever smaller storage as you use it. Finally, store therapeutic herbs out of the reach of children, just as you would with any commercial medication. Herbals can be potent stuff, and it's still unclear whether children should be using even reduced doses of herbal medications like St. John's Wort.

Could making homemade St. John's Wort remedies ever be really dangerous?

It's never wise to attempt self-medicating at all, and to do so with a "medicine" you make yourself adds to the risks. *Always* get a medical doctor's advice on whether your homegrown therapy is indicated or could be hazardous. It might be dangerous simply to waste time on experiments with St. John's Wort, commercial or homemade, if you are too ill for this treatment to be effective or have a condition for which it is not appropriate. You will have lost weeks you could have spent working with another, more effective therapy. For seriously depressed people or those with a condition that's just mimicking depression, that time can be critical. However, if you must experiment with homemade concoctions of an herb, there are certainly far more inherently dangerous plants you could be dealing with than St. John's Wort. Be assured that every herb is not so innocent. Just because it's found in nature doesn't mean something is safe. Belladonna is an oft-cited example. In the wrong amounts—easy to mistake when you're harvesting on your own—even a beneficial medicinal plant can become deadly. Homemade remedies made from other herbs have proven fatal when amateur herbalists have harvested the wrong plant by mistake. I found a recent report on a couple who died when the "comfrey" they harvested and ate turned out to be the foxglove instead. Even the comfrey could have had toxic effects with long-term use.

I'm a little nervous about using homemade medicinals. Is there anything I can do to make this process safer?

If you're nervous, why use a homemade therapy? Find a reputable commercial brand you can trust and stick with that. Still, if you verify the identity of your plant as St. John's Wort, avoid contaminated plants, have established you are not allergic to the herb, and are careful in your production, safety should not be a real issue in the case of St. John's Wort—in normal doses. If that sounds like a qualified response, that's because it is. Even exercise can be dangerous if it isn't done properly, so making your own medicines certainly carries a risk. As an added safeguard, scrutinize your physical and mental well-being when on this herbal remedy or any other therapy for side effects and benefits. Keep a journal recording doses, information from your remedy labels, and any changes you notice in your daily functioning, good or bad. Keep your doctors updated on the information in your records. If you refuse to get medical help and guidance—NOT a smart idea—at least tell family and friends what you're doing so they can inform medical personnel in case of severe toxic or allergic reactions. These reactions appear to be rare in the case of St. John's Wort, but are still a possibility, especially if you are growing your own or buying from a less-than-knowledgeable source. Mistakes can happen even to experts.

NINE

❧

Resource Section:
Depression and Alternative Medicine

Periodically in these pages you have encountered suggestions for taking your fact-finding mission beyond this book. That won't be as difficult as you may believe, because there is actually a wealth of information out there simply waiting for you to tap into it. In this section, you'll find ways to make connections that will help you focus your search: lists of organizations that may supply materials, referrals or support; web-site addresses for directing your on-line surfing sessions; and some reading suggestions for your next library or bookstore crawl. No single book can answer all the questions you have about how St. John's Wort can fit into your depression therapy, but with these resources, you'll be able to take your exploration of this herbal remedy to the next level.

Helpful Organizations

This listing will provide you with the basics on organizations and foundations dedicated to helping the depression sufferer. The services they provide vary, from supplying informational materials, to sponsoring educational programs, to connecting you with networks of doctors or fellow mood-disorder sufferers. The organizations featured here are just a few of those out there focusing on depression or alternative medicines and acting as caring patient advocates. These were

277

chosen for their reputation, longevity, and quality of information provided. Others you encounter may not be as reputable. Be cautious when approaching any organization you haven't heard good things about. Ask how current is their information and check with the Better Business Bureau in the area to see whether any reports have been filed against the organization. Use your instincts and your wits.

National Institutes of Health (NIH)

A part of the U.S. Department of Health and Human Services (DHHS), the NIH is actually a collection of twenty-four individual "institutes," located in seventy-five buildings, each dedicated to a particular field of medicine. The goals and mission for each of these institutes and for NIH as a whole is to discover and disseminate information on a wide range of health issues. It sponsors federal and nongovernmental research into all aspects of medical science, including mental health and alternative therapies. (See entries below.) The goal of this research, according to the NIH, is to "acquire new knowledge to help prevent, detect, diagnose, and treat disease and disability, from the rarest genetic disorder to the common cold." Two of the NIH branches include the National Institute for Mental Health and the Office of Alternative Medicine.

To support the research of these and its other divisions, the NIH maintains hospitals and research centers and the National Library of Medicine, a collection of 5 million medical books, journals, pamphlets, rare manuscripts, films, and other items comprising the world's largest medical library, called the "Fort Knox of health information."

National Institute for Mental Health (NIMH)

National Institute of Mental Health
NIMH Public Inquiries
5600 Fishers Lane, Room 7C-02, MSC 8030
Bethesda, MD 20892-8030
(301) 443-4513
http://www.nimh.nih.gov/home.htm

The NIMH is one of the arms of the National Institutes of Health which focuses on the subject of mental health, including, of course, mood disorders of every type. Its on-line site provides informative facts and research findings on mental illness, as well as statistics on its financial cost to the country. A few of the documents it currently provides (available on-line) include:

- Questions and answers about St. John's Wort
- Information on specific mental disorders, their diagnosis and treatment (in English and Spanish versions)
- Mental illness in America

The NIMH offers such informative publications to the public, education programs in anxiety disorders and depression, funds research, and is cosponsoring, along with the Library of Congress, the "Project on the Decade of the Brain," a public-awareness initiative on mental health continuing through the year 2000.

Most importantly, for depression sufferers interested in St. John's Wort, the NIMH's Psychotherapeutic Medication Program was created to support the evaluation of what it terms "orphan" treatments—those which could have tremendous impact on the public's health, but which do not have the support of corporate backers. It is this arm of the NIMH that is helping to fund the clinical trial now being conducted in the U.S. on the herbal remedy. It recently approved the proposal submitted by Duke University Medical Center (see below), which will be coordinating the trial.

The Office of Alternative Medicine (OAM)

OAM Information Center
Office of Alternative Medicine, NIH
9000 Rockville Pike, Room 5B-38
Bethesda, MD 20892
Telephone: (301) 402-2466
Fax: (301) 402-4741
FAX Board: (301) 402-2466
http://altmed.od.nih.gov/oam/
National Hotline Number: (800) 531-1794

The Office of Alternative Medicine (OAM) was created in 1992 and is an office of the National Institutes of Health

(NIH). According to the OAM, the Office "facilitates research and evaluation of unconventional medical practices and disseminates this information to the public." To support this, it provides a public-information clearinghouse of data relating to the subject of alternative therapies and funds research programs for the study of these treatments. The OAM does not, however, recommend referrals to individual alternative practitioners.

Duke University Medical Center

A university hospital, Duke University Medical Center has been given the NIMH grant to conduct a clinical trial on St. John's Wort for its treatment of mild to moderate depression. The study, which was assigned to Duke University Medical Center in the fall of 1997, will continue for approximately three years, monitoring patients during an acute phase of the trial and then a follow-up period. Together these phases will last six months. Over 300 patients will be studied at the university and up to 10 satellite medical centers around the country. Data will be reviewed and collected for another two years until released. Coordinators of the trial, which is being headed by Dr. Davidson, and doctors associated with it plan to be evaluating volunteers for the trial beginning summer of 1998. If you are interested in becoming involved in the trial, have your doctor contact Dr. Davidson at:

Duke University
Duke University Medical Center
Durham, NC 27706
(919) 684-8111

Bastyr University

145000 Juanita Drive Northeast
Bothell, WA 98011
(425) 823-1300
FAX: (425) 823-6222

Bastyr is a twenty-year-old nonprofit institution for the study of alternative and natural medicine, and the only regionally accredited education and research center with this focus located in the United States. Graduates can receive a doctorate in naturopathic medicine, an approach that promotes the use of plant-based therapies, a master of science in nutrition, acupuncture, or acupuncture and Oriental medicine. Students can also receive a master of arts in applied behavioral sciences. A well-respected university that has received a landmark grant from the OAM, Bastyr is a forerunner in the study of alternative treatments. It would be a good place to start your search for an alternative practitioner if you are unable to obtain a referral from a friend, physician, or someone else whose opinion you trust. Call its alumni office and ask if any graduates of the university have a practice near you.

Here are some organizations that can help you find or establish mental illness support groups in your area:

Depression after Delivery

P.O. Box 1282
Morrisville, PA 19067
(215) 295-3994 or (800) 944-4773

A national organization formed of approximately 100 affiliated groups, Depression after Delivery provides support for women who are experiencing postpartum depression with phone contacts, newsletters, conferences, and programs, and by connecting women with others with the same disorder.

Postpartum Support International

927 N. Kellogg Avenue
Santa Barbara, CA 93111
(805) 967-7636 (during the daytime, in PST)

This organization was also developed to spread the word on postpartum depression—its diagnosis and treatment. It can offer referral and connect you to groups in your area, or help you begin one.

Depressed Anonymous International

> P.O. Box 17471
> Louisville, KY 40217
> (502) 569-1989
> E-mail: depanon@aol.com

Utilizing the classic 12-step approach, this organization is a support group that offers workshops, seminars, newsletters, phone support, referrals, and information materials.

National Depressive and Manic-Depressive Association

> 730 N. Franklin, Suite 501
> Chicago, IL 60610
> (800) 826-3632 or (312) 642-0049
> FAX: (312) 642-7243
> http://www.ndmda.org

A national organization of nearly 300 chapters, this association supplies informational and emotional support to people diagnosed as bipolar and to their families.

Mood Disorders Support Group, Inc. (MDSG-NY) Model Group

> P.O. Box 1747
> Madison Square Station
> New York, NY 10159
> (212) 533-MDSG
> FAX: (212) 475-5109

Both bipolar and depressive patients should contact this organization if they are interested in starting a support group in their own area. MDSG will supply information on how to get started, and connect patients to guest lectures and discussion groups.

Depression and Related Affective Disorders Association (DRADA)

Meyer 3-181 600 N. Wolfe Street
Baltimore, MD 21287-7381
(410) 955-4647 (daytime)
FAX: (410) 614-3241

This association provides assistance to those with depression and bipolar disorders, by supporting self-help groups, disseminating information, and sponsoring research and educational programs. Two such programs include: the Young People's Outreach Project and the Depression in the Workplace Project.

Recovery, Inc.

Over 800 affiliated groups provide support for self-help treatment of the feelings of depression, anxiety, nervousness, anger, and fear. The groups focus on a behavioral-change approach to mood disturbances.

Recovery, Inc.
802 N. Dearborn Street
Chicago, IL 60610
(312) 337-5661
FAX: (312) 337-5756
http://www.recovery-inc.com

O.C. Foundation, Inc.

Box 70
Milford, CT 06460-0070
(203) 878-5669 (during daytimes) or (203) 874-3843 (for a recorded message)
FAX: (203) 874-2826
E-mail: jphs28a@prodigy.com
http://pages.prodigy.com/alwillen/ocf.html and also through a bulletin board on the Prodigy service provider; look for postings under the heading Depression/Anxiety/OCD

National Organization for Seasonal Affective Disorder (NOSAD)

P.O. Box 40190
Washington, DC 20016
A nationwide association dedicated to sharing information
about this disorder.

Other organizations that can help with information about mood
disorders:

National Mental Health Association

1021 Prince Street
Alexandria, VA 22314
(880) 969-NMHA

National Foundation for Depressive Illness

P.O. Box 2257
New York, NY 10116
(800) 248-4344

National Alliance for the Mentally Ill (NAMI)

2101 Wilson Blvd., Suite 302
Arlington, VA 22201
(800) 950-NAMI

This organization also incorporates a Children and Adolescents' Network (NAMI: CAN) and Sibling and Adult Children's Network (NAMI: SAC) for the families of patients and young victims of mental illness.

Other organizations that can help with information about herbs:

American Botanical Council & HerbalGram

P.O. Box 201660
Austin, TX 78720

The council is dedicated to the dissemination of information on herbs and their applications. In order to generate the public and professional awareness of botanical products and herbal remedies, it produces the often-cited journal *HerbalGram* in cooperation with the Herb Research Foundation. *HerbalGram* contains articles by researchers and scientists on the current explorations of plant therapies.

Herb Research Foundation

1007 Pearl Street, Suite 200
Boulder, CO 80302
(303) 449-2265
FAX: (303) 449-7849
http://sunsite.unc.edu/herbs

A wealth of information is provided by this organization on herbs and their therapies, chemistry, analysis, and history— much of it available online. See information about *Herbal-Gram*, above.

American Herb Association

P.O. Box 1673
Nevada City, CA 95959

A respected organization with members who exchange information via newsletters. These include late-breaking news about herb and other botanicals, research into their applications, legal challenges, articles, and Q&As. Write for a pamphlet describing membership.

American Herbalist Guild

Box 1683
Soquel, CA 95073

An association of professional herbalists, this would be a good source for referrals of herbal practitioners in your area; ask for as much information as you can from the organization and from the herbalists to which it refers you.

American Association of Naturopath Physicians

2366 Eastlake Avenue East, Suite 322
Seattle, WA 98102
FAX: (206) 323-7621
http://inifinite.org/Naturopathic.Physician

This organization will provide you with a list of its members; the site offers general health information. When contacting a local practitioner, you should ask for referrals from patients who would feel comfortable talking with you about their care. Be sure to ask if the ND is licensed by the state if that applies (only eleven states license these practitioners: Alaska, Arizona, Connecticut, Hawaii, Maine, Montana, New Hampshire, Oregon, Utah, Vermont, Washington) and has graduated from an accredited school such as Bastyr University.

Useful INTERNET Locations

Some terms to know:

- *URL*—the "address" where a site can be found, pictured in a window at the top of your on-screen window. URLs get longer and more complicated the deeper into a site you go, so it's often easier to type in the home-page address and then click on to new pages from there
- *Link*—connections to other web sites provided by a given page; when clicked, links will automatically forward you to the new site without your having to type in a new address. Links are usually indicated on a page by underlining a word that relates to the new site, or by highlighting text in another color
- *Home page*—the first page in a web site, it usually gives or links you to pages describing the person or organization maintaining the material and acts like a table of contents to the rest of the site

The first question many people have about information they find on-line dealing with health issues is a basic one: Is it reliable? The answer is less simple and straightforward: It depends. It depends on who is providing the information, why they offer it, and how recently it was posted. Many people have only good intentions when sharing their interests and opinions on the Internet, but the truth is, they all can say what they like and anyone can sound like an expert. Written words can appear to carry weight, but it's up to you to do a little digging to find out how much of the authority you grant them is actually deserved.

The sites listed below are some that are reputable and informative. Try them first, then use the instructions for searching the web to find some more. The information posted on these sites at the time of this writing was both informative and broad-ranging enough not to seem too partisan. But the Internet is a very changeable and evolving entity. When you visit links provided by these sites or that you encounter elsewhere, do a little investigating to find out who's actually providing the information you are reading: Go to the home page of a site—this is generally accessible via a link on each page, but it can also be found by trimming the URL down to its bare bones in the address window. The home page is the place to look for information about who's doing the posting and when it was last updated. Beware of commercial sites; they occasionally masquerade as educational sites. While they can provide interesting or entertaining information to back up their pitches, the material is typically one-sided at best, or downright false in the worst-case scenarios. My advice is to make notes about what you've found and copy or download pages to take with you on your next visit to the doctor. Don't take what you read there as gospel, but use it to start a dialogue with your physician, who can help you sort fact from fiction.

Here are some tips on sites to try that will help direct your next on-line session:

Search Words
You could spend a lot of time and effort trying to track down good sites and typing in their addresses, hoping you've typed them in correctly or that they are available through the service provider or connection you're using to access the Internet. Better still for the Internet surfer are the variety of "search engines" offered for free on-line, where the labor of finding and cataloguing sites has already been done. Ask anyone familiar with the web and she'll reel off a favorite search engine. Some

of the most popular general-interest engines include: Excite, Yahoo, WebCrawler, and Altavista. You'll find information on a lesser-known but incredibly helpful search engine below, Northern Light. There are also more subject-focused engines, such as the scientifically minded MedLine, but these frequently charge for the full-text versions of articles they hunt down or are available only to fee-paying members.

Once in a search engine you feel comfortable using, you would enter "search words" that tell the search engine what subjects it should look for information about in its files of millions of sites. The simple search word "depression" will net you an unbelievable number of "hits" during an on-line search, many of them containing little or no information of value on the subject you're really interested in finding out about. A search for "herb" will net you a lot of "hits" that, when followed, will take you to sites about someone named Herb. To get the most out of your time on-line, target and refine your search as much as possible using carefully chosen search words. Here are some combinations you might try:

> depression +herbs +alternative medicine
> "Saint John's Wort" +depression +NIMH study
> *Hypericum* +constituents
> Hypericin +AIDS
> *Hypericum perforatum* −sale (you might use the negative sign in front of this word if you were trying to weed out commercial sites)

Sometimes the word AND or NOT is used instead of the plus or negative sign; often it's simply a matter of preference; just be careful not to leave a space between the sign and the word it is defining. Placing a phrase in quotes means you'd like the search engine to look for the words together as a complete phrase. For instance, "Saint John's Wort" tells the engine to look for the herb and not call up sites about the individual words in the phrase, netting you sites on a variety of saints. The more definitive and subject-specific your language, the better off you'll be. In a search of St. John's Wort, then, you might choose the Latin term *"Hypericum"* as your base search term instead of the more common name for the herb. This will help eliminate many commercial sites, where the Latin isn't used, and will call up some scientific sites that do not use the common term. Even with careful search words, your hits will range from spot-on to wildly off-base. Be patient. Try other word combinations, or find one site that's close to what you are looking for and click on options offering to search for others like it.

Finally, a word of warning: A lot of information found online is not accurate or even truthful. Even reputable sites may not have access to the most recent information and still be passing along older, less accurate information, despite the relative "newness" of the technology. Check for dates on the page to find out when the information was posted. And keep in mind that on-line sites and the people you encounter there cannot diagnose your illness or attempt to predict how you will react to a treatment. The most important thing to keep in mind when wandering the web: On-line information is never intended to take the place of the doctor/patient relationship. Only a physician familiar with *your* unique expression of a disorder, *your* family history and current life situation, and *your* overall health can make an accurate diagnosis and suggest therapies tailored to you.

Northern Light
http://www.nlsearch.com

This search engine is a true find. It refines explorations on any subject but is especially helpful when you are attempting to wade through the depths of medical information out there. In addition to a database similar to that of other search engines, Northern Light has two million sites that are exclusive to the engine—some of these require a fee, but the vast majority are free. Each hit is listed with a brief entry that provides a helpful summary of the site (a little more informative than that of most search engines), the address of the site, and often the date of the posting. The entries also classify sites by general category such as "government site," "personal page," or "educational site," and let you know whether the information on it is free (designated by the flag "WW") or requires a fee ("special collection"). The fee pages are usually only a few dollars to download; information about becoming a Northern Lights member is provided—membership allows you a finite number of free downloads each month. However, most of the hits will not require any such outlay. Once a search is complete, hits are listed in the usual closest-match first, least-direct last. But the page also helpfully organizes information into subcategories that will help you further refine your search. Some categories pulled out from the *"Hypericum"* and *"depression"* searches included:

- Special Collection documents—documents for which there is a fee (generally $1), often newspapers, medical journals, or other copyrighted materials exclusive to the search engine
- Commercial sites—these are sites maintained by companies selling products related to the subject matter, in this case herbal remedies or books on the subjects of St. John's Wort, herbs, or depression
- www.hypericum.com—a link to the definitive web source for information on St. John's Wort (See more on this site below.)
- Vitamins
- Prozac
- Dietary supplements
- Antidepressant drugs
- AIDS and AIDS-related complications
- Herbs
- Personal pages—this category includes pages posted by universities and individuals
- Government sites

Sites with Drug Information

PharmInfoNet:
http://pharminfo.com
Health*touch*®:
http://www.healthtouch.com
RxList:
http://www.rxlist.com
These sites provide a variety of ways for you to search for material on prescription drugs and the illnesses they treat: databases that let you look for information on a drug using either its generic or brand name; indexes of articles about individual drugs as well as press releases by pharmaceutical and biotech-

nology industries on their products (you'll find information about some of the newest drugs being tested there but the information may be biased); and answers to frequently asked questions about drugs culled from a variety of sources, including pharmacy services, pharmaceutical companies, and medical professionals. Some also feature brief articles about drug-related subjects and links to illness-specific sites.

Sites with Herbal or Alternative Medicine Information

Hypericum and Depression
http://www.hypericum.com/toc.htm
Any search of *"Hypericum"* on the web will take you to this site, a generous outpouring from Harold H. Bloomfield, MD, Mikael Nordfors, MD, and Peter McWilliams, authors of the best-selling title by that name. It contains the complete text of their book, published in 1996. Although some of the information from the book is now dated (yes, that's how quickly medical innovations can happen), the authors continue to update their material via on-line addendums. The site covers some history of the herb and its application as an antidepressant, and summarizes some of the studies done.

FAQ on St. John's Wort
http://www.primenet.com/~camilla/STJOHNS.FAQ
If you visit only one site on-line for information about St. John's Wort, this would probably be it. It is a one-stop-shopping FAQ (Frequently Asked Questions) on St. John's Wort that provides exceedingly up-to-date and thorough information on the herb, in a format that is briefer and perhaps easier to absorb than the much larger hypericum.com site. Maintained by Camilla Cracchiolo, a registered nurse, it covers the basics from the herb's many uses, antidepressant effects, safety, side effects, possible drug interactions, and chemical constituents: a definitive resource on the herb.

Southwest School of Botanical Medicine
http://www.chili.rt66.com/hrbmoore/HOMEPAGE
An oft-cited, expansive site of all things herbal: archives of ancient illustrations and modern photographs of herbs; lists of plants by genus, species, location, and other searchable in-

dexes; classic works in botanical medicine including excerpts and complete texts from a variety of herbal *Materia Medicas*; abstracts of studies and research conducted into herbal remedies; links to other herb sites; and numerous manuals and folios written by Michael Moore, director of the 20-year-old school and a well-respected herbalist.

Henriette's Herbal Homepage
http://www.sunsite.unc.edu/herbmed
This page, maintained by Henriette Kress, has some time-saving links to sites with herbal information and also provides a cataloging of information you'll find scattered piecemeal elsewhere, such as FAQs (Frequently Asked Questions) generated from queries found on herbal newsgroups, organized by subject. This site also links you to databases of plant names and archives of herb pictures that will help you identify your samples and to other herb-centered sites (such as the Southwest School's home page, described previously).

> *http://www.wellnessadvocate.com*
> *http://www.botanical.com*
> *http://www.all-natural.com*
> *http://www.healthyideas.com*
> *http://home.miningco.com/health*

These are noncommercial sites with a focus on alternative medicines, herbs or both. They provide some basic background on the St. John's Wort and other herbal remedies, including botanical names, genus and species lists, folklore, links to other herbal sites such as botanical gardens and societies, Q&As, book lists, and connections to chat rooms and usegroups. Keep in mind that the information in sites such as these or their extended links is not always accurate or especially current. As always, take anything you read on the web with a grain of salt. The Mining Company site, which is nothing like what its name suggestions, also boasts an ''herbs for health'' link that will take you to a very thorough FAQ on St. John's Wort.

The Alternative Medicine Home page
http://www.pitt.edu/~cbw/altm.html
This page describes itself as "a jumpstation for sources of information on unconventional, unorthodox, unproved, or alternative, complementary, innovative, integrative therapies." You can find a variety of links to sites both authoritative and off the beaten path.

Sites with General Medical and Mood Disorder Information

Psycom.Net
http://www.psycom.net/
This site is of value for its link to the *International Journal of Psychopathology, Psychotherapy and Psychopharmacology* (for the medically trained) but primarily for its connection to *Dr. Ivan's Depression Central*. Depression Central is an extraordinary find for someone suffering from a mood disorder. It contains links to literally dozens of other sites and source materials, covering the gamut from major depression, bipolar disorder, dysthymia, and other mood disorders. It describes itself as the "Internet's central clearinghouse for information on all types of depressive disorders and on the most effective treatments for individuals suffering from them," and that's just what it is. It will save you untold hours of searching and covers a broad spectrum of information even within those mood disorder categories. Here are just a few of the links you'll find there. Each of these leads to pages focusing even more specifically on the subject, giving guidelines for finding good treatment, finding out more, Q&As, etc:

Begin here to Read About Mood Disorders	Bipolar (Manic-Depressive) Disorder	Books and Videos about Depressive Disorders
Borderline Personality Disorder	Borna virus-induced Depression	
Causes of Mood Disorders	Combined Drug Treatment and Psychotherapy	Cyclothymia

Depression in Children and Adolescents

Depression in the Elderly

Depression in Special Populations

Diagnosis and Classification of Depression

Drug Treatment for People with Mood Disorders

Dysthymia

Electroconvulsive Therapy (ECT)

Epidemiology of Mood Disorders

Famous People with Mood Disorders

For the Friends and Families of People with Mood Disorders

Genetics of Depressive Illnesses

Grief and bereavement

HIV and Depression

Hospitals—The Best Psychiatric Hospitals

Manic-Depression

Major (Unipolar) Depression

New York City Mood Disorders Support Group (MDSG/NY)

Postpartum Depressions

Premenstrual Dysphoria

Psychiatrists Specializing in the Treatment of People with Mood Disorders

Mood Disorders

Psychotherapy for People with Depression Accepting Volunteers

Research Studies in NYC Accepting Volunteers

Research Studies at the NIMH (Bethesda, Maryland)

Research Study at UCLA Accepting Volunteers

Schizoaffective Disorder

Screening for Depressive Illness

Search MEDLINE at No Cost

Digital Librarian: a librarian's choice of the best of the web

http://www.servtech.com/public/mvail/health.html

This site, maintained by a librarian named Margaret Vail Anderson, provides links to a remarkably comprehensive list of health and science sites. You'll find connections to every kind of medical location on the web, from universities, organizations, government addresses, personal pages, and commercial sites; each is given a brief description that can help you fine-tune your next leap.

HealthWorld Online

http://www.healthy.net/

This site is another clearinghouse of links to valuable information. In addition to providing tips for finding qualified herbal practitioners, lists of educational foundations and professional associations, trade journal and consumer magazine connections and book lists, and addresses for laboratory services for testing herbal preparations, the site gives you information on these subjects (among others):

Alternative Medicine	Integrating Alternative and Mainstream Medicine
Alternative Approaches to Specific Health Conditions	Alternative Medicine Discussion Forums
Alternative Medicine Resource Center	Systems of Traditional Medicine
Acupuncture	Ayurvedic Medicine
Chiropractic	Herbal Medicine
Homeopathy	Naturopathic Medicine
Osteopathy	Traditional Chinese Medicine
Alternative Therapies	Aromatherapy
Biofeedback Training	Bodywork and Somatic Therapies
Chelation Therapy	
Energy Medicine/Bio-Energetic Medicine	Detoxification Therapies
	Environmental Medicine
Fasting	Flower Remedies
Guided Imagery	Holistic Dentistry
Mind/Body Medicine	Nutritional (Orthomolecular) Medicine
Qigong (Chi Kung) and Taiji (Tai Chi)	

Mental Health Net
http://www.cmhc.com/
A truly helpful site for those interested in or suffering from mood disorders is the Mental Health Net, sponsored by CMHC. The very accessible site is both a search engine and an information address, supplying brief clips on latest mental-health news and providing a guide to over 7,000 individual resources on the web that deal with the diagnosis and treatment of mental illnesses including: depression, anxiety, panic attacks, chronic fatigue syndrome, and substance abuse. It also offers links to professional journals and self-help magazines.

The site hooks up to on-line databases, suggests books and other materials that are helpful, provides hints for working within managed-care systems, lists support-group organizations, and has forums for on-line discussions.

Sites with AIDS Information (also contains general health information)

Critical Path AIDS Project
http://www.critpath.org/
This is a tremendously helpful web site, and one that would be useful not just to AIDS patients but to anyone interested in alternative therapy. The site provides lists of and links to alternative-medicine organizations and many botanical pages providing information on herbs and their preparation as well as other alternative systems. This site can save you time hunting around for these often difficult-to-find addresses. And, of course, it is an exhaustive clearinghouse for data about the most current AIDS-HIV treatments, research, support groups and organizations and referrals to regional services.

Sites Where you Can "Talk" with Other Mood Disorder Sufferers

Newsgroups
Deja News
http://www.dejanews.com
(Or do a search for "herbs +newsgroups" and your engine should guide you)

Chatrooms

Michael Tierra's PlanetHerbs On-line Forum
http://www.planetherbs.com/forum/goforum.html

Algy's Herb Talk
http://www.algy.com/herb/index.html.

Ethnobotany Cafe Bulletin Board
http://countrylife.net/ethnobotany/main.html

(Or look for links to subject-related chat rooms found attached to informational sites; you can try entering "chat rooms" on your search engine and following those links but it is often difficult to find rooms focusing on medical subjects that way)

America Online

If you are on America Online, a prolonged pursuit can lead you to a wonderful array of scheduled chat sessions on very specific topics relating to mood disorder, including depression recovery; panic/anxiety on-line mutual support depressive disorders; mental health seminars; behind the scenes: the mental health system and you; obsessive-compulsive disorder self-help, mental health and bipolar disorder mutual support and more. Begin at the AOL category "health" and work your way through various mental health pathways to reach a schedule. AOL also has chat groups on alternative medicines. Start in the same "health" location and travel through Altmed: Alternative Medicine Focus to reach the chat rooms.

In addition to providing educational sites, the Internet can also be of value by connecting you to other people experiencing a similar daily struggle with depression—or from whatever mood disorder you may have. The best places to "meet" people who share your problem is in "Usenet newsgroups" or "chat rooms." For people who cannot attend support groups for their disorder—either through bashfulness, ill health, or an isolated location—on-line conversations or exchanges with other sufferers can be a lifesaver. Patients discover they aren't alone and that, in fact, complete strangers will care deeply about their recovery and offer to help. The usual cautions apply, of course—don't share identifying personal information about yourself or provide names and addresses unless you are as sure as you can be about the credibility the person with whom you are "speaking." Remember, the information you find in newsgroups and chat rooms is, despite its good intent, often inaccurate. The best way to use material you find in these places is as a stepping-stone for discussions with your own doctor.

Usenet newsgroups perform a function similar to that of community bulletin boards, albeit for very focused communities. You may post or answer questions on virtually any subject—there are herbal newsgroups and those which focus on depression, anxiety disorders, or alternative medicine. Some newsgroups allow you to exchange this information in real time; that is, people respond to your message as soon as you post it. Some newsgroups sites are sponsored by commercial sites, but many are provided by universities, informational organizations, or even individuals with an intense interest in the subject.

Here are some of the newsgroups found when a search for "herbs" was made in the Deja News newsgroup site:

- alt.folklore.herbs (something of a misnomer, as it covers all facts of herbal medicine, not just folklore)
- misc.health.alternative
- alt.support.depression
- soc.support.depression.treatment
- alt.support.anxiety
- alt.support.survivors
- alt.drugs.psychedelic
- alt.support.menopause
- alt.support.dissociat
- bit.listserv.autism
- alt.support.attn-defi
- alt.support.skin-dise Ed

A form of real-time exchange also occurs in chat rooms. In these "rooms" you can join ongoing discussion groups about a variety of subjects. Although chat rooms sometimes have very specific themes, described by their names, conversations may become quite casual and meander off the subject. This can be frustrating for people who want quick, direct answers and a very focused exchange, but it can be a boon to sufferers looking to connect with people who have the same mood-disorder background, and who might see things from a similar, illness-defined viewpoint, but who don't necessarily want to talk about their condition at length. Chat room conversations are occasionally organized ahead of time for a prescheduled day and time, to discuss a very specific topic. These often feature a "guest appearance" by an expert in the field and are usually conducted under the aegis of a site manager, who directs and monitors the conversation.

Books

Herbal

The Honest Herbal, by Varro E. Tyler. 1993

Home Herbal, by Penelope Ody. 1995

Pocket Medicinal Herbs, by Penelope Ody. 1997

Herbs: An Illustrated Encyclopedia, by Kathie Keville. 1994

The Encyclopedia of Medicinal Plants, by Andrew Chevallier. 1996

The Herb Book, by John Lust. 1974

On Mental Illness

Listening to Prozac, by Peter D. Kramer. 1993

Beyond Prozac, by Michael J. Norden, M.D. 1996

APPENDIX A

Making Measurements Easier to Understand

Since many medicines base their quantities on the metric system, American consumers can be bewildered by the unfamiliar amounts they see listed on packages. And amateur herbalists will find that many of the traditional guides for preparing remedies list ingredients using metric standards as well. Here you'll find some measurement equivalencies that should make your shopping for St. John's Wort less confusing.

Remember, the metric system is based on powers of ten and metric prefixes are applied to the base term "gram" for weight and "liter" to measure fluid volume, so . . .

IF YOU SEE THE PREFIX	MULTIPLY THE BASE BY
Deka	10
Hecto	100
Deci	0.10 (it means a tenth of)
Centi	0.01 (it means a hundredth of)
Milli	0.001 (it means a thousandth of)
Micro	0.0001 (it means a millionth of)

What if you have a prescription or recipe measured in one system and want to find its equivalent in another system? Here are some tips:

YOU'VE GOT ONE	TO FIND OUT HOW MANY	YOU MUST MULTIPLY BY
dry ounce by weight (oz)	grams (g)	28
gram	dry ounces	0.035
milligram (mg)	ounces	0.000035
fluid ounce by volume (oz)	milliliters (ml)	30
milliliter	ounces	0.34
pint (p)	liters (l)	0.47
liter	pints	2.1
quart (qt)	liters	0.95
liter	quarts	1.06
teaspoon (tsp)	milliliters	4.93
tablespoon (tbs)	milliliters	14.79
cup	liters	0.24

* equivalents will be approximate

Here are some other equivalents you may run across in depression therapies:

ONE OF THESE	= ONE OF THESE
fluid dram aka drachm	= 1/8 fluid ounce
dry ounce by weight	= 8 drams
dry ounce by weight	= 480 grains
dry dram by weight	= 60 grains
fluid ounce	= 29.5 cubic centimeters
British fluid ounce	= 28.4 cubic centimeters (cc)
British imperial quart	= 1.200095 U.S. quarts
teaspoon	= approximately 1 fluid dram or 4 cubic centimeters
dessert spoon	= approximately 2 fluid drams or 8 cubic centimeters
tablespoon	= approximately 1/2 ounce or 16 cubic centimeters
British teaspoon	= approximately 5 cubic centimeters

British tablespoon = approximately 15 cubic centimeters

gram = 20 drops (according to the generally recognized standard determined by distilled water; but drops are notoriously erratic measures—depending on the size of the dispenser's aperture, there can be as few as 40 and as many as 170 or more drops per fluid dram)

And, just to make things really confusing—the same terms are used in prescription writing in both the U.S. and some European countries, but the weights they measure can be different. U.S. pharmacies still tend to use the apothecaries' system. Countries using weights standardized by the British Pharmacopoeia use what's known as the avoirdupois system. The weight of the grain is the same in both systems, but it's downhill from there. Here's how the two differ:

THE U.S. PHARMACOPOEIA

1 pound =	12 ounces =	96 drams =	5760 grains

THE BRITISH PHARMACOPOEIA

1 pound =	16 ounces =	256 drams =	7000 grains

APPENDIX B

What's on the Shelves

Name of product	What it is	Who makes it	What general information the manufacturer gives you
St. John's Wort Tea	tea	The Yogi Tea Company	St. John's Wort historical background . . . the company's toll-free number and web-site address . . . warning against use during pregnancy . . . directions for making tea . . . suggested dose . . . satisfaction guarantee . . . yoga exercise tip
St. John's Wort Tea Bags	tea	Alvita (A Twinlab Division)	a partial company address . . . background on the company . . . environmental-concern claims
Hypericum Verbatim	tablet	Hypericum Buyers Club	how to adjust dosages with the scored tablet

The claims	Herb and/or hypericin content (if provided) *indicates sold in a variety of herb/hypericin combinations	What else is in there	Number of doses (for adult in prime) and average cost (may not include shipping)
"St. John's Wort Tea is formulated to bring balance to those who experience mood swings"	850 mg of St. John's Wort (no hypericin content given) per bag	fennel seed, spearmint leaf, organic cinnamon bark, clove bud, ginger root, black pepper, lavender flowers, cardamom seed, fenugreek seed and natural flavor (caffeine-free)	16 bags (5–8 days' use at their suggested dosing) @ $4.00
references to unspecified "health benefits"	No content information provided	no content information provided	24 bags (no suggested dosages provided) @ $3.00
mood stabilizer	300 mg with 0.3% hypericin per tablet	inactive ingredients	280 tablets 1/day @ $29.00

Name of product	What it is	Who makes it	What general information the manufacturer gives you
St. John's Wort	capsule	Solaray	historical background; general information on benefits; pregnancy warning
St. John's Power	capsule	Nature's Herbs	historical information; scientific claims; pregnancy warning; fair skin and photosensitivity warning
St. John's Wort	capsule	Nature's Sunshine	historical information; disclaimer about medicinal claims made elsewhere by manufacturer; generalized study results

The claims	Herb and/or hypericin content (if provided) *indicates sold in a variety of herb/hypericin combinations	What else is in there	Number of doses (for adult in prime) and average cost (may not include shipping)
intended to provide dietary support to help maintain healthy central nervous system	300 mg with 0.3% hypericin*	inactive ingredients; hawthorn berries, cellulose, stearic acid, silica	60 capsules 1–3/day with meal or water @ $11.00
"just as helpful as commonly used drugs, without side effects such as headaches and vomiting" [website]	standardized extract of 90/300 mg with 0.3% hypericin*	antioxidants	120 capsules (1 capsule 3 times/day) @ $20.49
"documented research supports St. John Wort's usage for depression and slowing growth of the AIDS virus"	300 mg with 1 mg hypericin	passionflower	100 capsules (33 days' use at their suggested dosing) @ $26.50

Name of product	What it is	Who makes it	What general information the manufacturer gives you
Depress-Ex	capsules (Vegi-caps®)	Crystal Star	
St. John's Wort	capsules	Jarrow Formulas	
Positive Thoughts	tablets	Source Naturals	lists some constituents
St. John's Wort	tablets	Source Naturals	

The claims	Herb and/or hypericin content (if provided) *indicates sold in a variety of herb/hypericin combinations	What else is in there	Number of doses (for adult in prime) and average cost (may not include shipping)
		kava, American ginseng root, ashwagandha, gotu kola, skullcap, Siberian ginseng root, rosemary leaf, wood betony, fo-ti, ginger root	90 capsules (22–45 days' use at their suggested dosing) @ $17.00
	300 mg. with 0.3% hypericin*		60 capsules 1/day @ $10.00
	900 mg with 0.3% hypericin, also listed as 2.7 mg hypericin	valerian root, kava root, lemon balm, GABA, taurine, magnesium, L-Tyrosine, N-Acetyl L-Tyrosine, L-Phenylalanine, DMAE, vitamin C, B_1, B_3, B_5, B_6, B_{12}, biotin, folic acid, manganese, zinc	90 tablets (1 tablet 3 times daily) between meals; allow 6 weeks for results @ $23.50
	300 mg. with 0.3% hypericin		120 tablets 1/day @ $19.25

Name of product	What it is	Who makes it	What general information the manufacturer gives you
St. John's Wort Extract	capsules	Nature's Way	historical information; how it's produced
St. John's Wort Extract	capsules	Optimal Nutrients	
St. John's Wort Whole Extract	Vegi-cap® capsules	Elixir Tonics & Teas	
Kira	tablet	Lichtwer Pharma U.S.	
Herbal Active	tablets	Nature's Plus	

The claims	Herb and/or hypericin content (if provided) *indicates sold in a variety of herb/hypericin combinations	What else is in there	Number of doses (for adult in prime) and average cost (may not include shipping)
"promotes a positive mad"	St. John's Wort Extract—150mg; St. John's Wort Herb—350mg; 0.3% hypericin*		100 capsules (1–2 twice a day); take with water between meals; use for 2 months @ $14.50
	300 mg. with 0.3% hypericin		120 capsules 1/day @ $17.00
"no animal products"	300 mg, 0.3% hypericin (from German extract)	tablet is coated with sugar	90 capsules @ $17.00
	300 mg, 0.3% hypericin (from German extract)		45 tablets @ $16.00
"greater activity than non-standard 300 mg" "MAOI properties"	250 mg with 0.3–0.5% hypericin		60 tablets, 1 per day @ $10.50

Name of product	What it is	Who makes it	What general information the manufacturer gives you
St. John's Wort	caplet	NuNaturals	disclaimer about medicinal claims made elsewhere by company;
St. John's Wort	capsule	Kombucha Power Products	lists constituents; lists parts of herb used, gives warnings to pregnant and lactating women; warns of photosensitivity
St. John's Wort Extract	capsules	Nature's Life	disclaimer about medical claims made elsewhere by company; warnings about photosensitivity; cautions to pregnant/lactating women and users of antidepressant drugs

The claims	Herb and/or hypericin content (if provided) *indicates sold in a variety of herb/hypericin combinations	What else is in there	Number of doses (for adult in prime) and average cost (may not include shipping)
"calming frayed nerves" "sleep better"	300 mg with 0.3% hypericin standardized	5 Hydroxy-tryptophan, Kava Kava	120 caplets, 1–3 daily @ $19.00
"recent studies have found this herb to be a safe, rational supplement for treating mild to moderate depression"	250 mg with 0.3% hypericin, also listed as 750 mcg hypericin		60 capsules, 1 per day @ $14.00
"helps improve mood and increase brain transmission"	300 mg with 0.3% hypericin, standardized		50 capsules, 1–2 per day @ $10.00

Name of product	What it is	Who makes it	What general information the manufacturer gives you
St. John's Wort	Vegi-cap® capsules	Elixir	the company's website provides historical information, brief summary of the clinical trials, other applications, and general guidelines for the use of St. John's Wort in depression therapy
Kira (Hypericum Tablets, aka St. John's Wort)	Tablets	Lichtwer Pharma	the package mentions Kira's use in Europe and suggests most benefit within four weeks. Via a toll-free phone line, you are given mostly vague claims. The message mentions that this formula is known as LI-160, but does not tell consumers that LI-160 is the extract used in many of the European clinical studies and is one of the prescription formulas available in Germany.

The claims	Herb and/or hypericin content (if provided) *indicates sold in a variety of herb/hypericin combinations	What else is in there	Number of doses (for adult in prime) and average cost (may not include shipping)
"research-grade Hypericum," "safe, natural alternative to prescription anti-depressants," "[Vegicaps] dissolve quickly in the alimentary tracts unlike gelatin capsules or tablets"	300 mg	no animal by-products or binder materials	90 Vegicaps® (their suggested dosing not known–I did not obtain sample) @ $17.00
"the only Hypericum supplement proven in extensive and on-going research to help you maintain a healthy emotional balance," "to improve your perspective, renew your confidence and get you back on track"	unknown	Contains no preservatives, yeast or gluten	45 tablets (9 days' use at their suggested dosing) @ $15.00

Name of product	What it is	Who makes it	What general information the manufacturer gives you
Hypericum Verbatim	Tablets	Hypericum Buyer's Club	this is research-grade Hypericum
St. John's Wort Herb Extract	Vegicaps	Solgar	photosensitivity warning; shouldn't be taken with tyramine-containing foods such as meats and cheeses; pregnancy/lactation warning
St. John's Wort with Kava	Capsules	TwinLab	general medical disclaimer; pregnancy warning; photosensitivity warning; sedative/tranquilizer will cause drowsiness
St. John's Wort	Capsules	Mason	

The claims	Herb and/or hypericin content (if provided) *indicates sold in a variety of herb/hypericin combinations	What else is in there	Number of doses (for adult in prime) and average cost (may not include shipping)
	300 mg	no animal products	280 tablets (90 days' use at their suggested dosing) @ $33.00 [Mail order only at 1-888-HYPERI-CUM (1-888-497-3742)]
	herb extract 175 mg; raw herb powder 300 mg; 0.3% hypericin. In a base of phyt0_2X; special blend of antioxidants maintain freshness of herbs by preventing oxidation		60 capsules (1–3 daily) preferably at mealtime @ $8.25
"mood booster and calming formula"	300 mg with 0.3% hypericin; 250 mg kava root extract		60 capsules (1 capsules 3 times a day) @ $10.99
"the uplifting herb promotes positive mood and feeling"	300 mg with 0.3% hypericin	dicalcium phosphate, gelatin, magnesium stearate	60 capsules (2 a day) @ $6.99

Bibliography

Adler M.; "Prediction: onset of improved mood after 2 weeks. Hypericum therapy in intermediate class depression." [German; English abstract] *Fortschritte Der Medizin* 1997 Aug 30; 115(24):49–50.

Algy's Herb Page @*http://www.algy.com/herb/index.html*.

Alsop R., editor and Wall Street Journal Editors; *The Wall Street Journal Almanac*, 1998. New York: Ballantine Books, Inc., 1997.

American Psychiatric Association; *Diagnostic and Statistical Manual of Mental Disorders*, 4th ed. (DSM IV). Washington, D.C., 1994.

American Psychiatric Association; "Practice guideline for the treatment of major depressive disorder in adults." *American Journal of Psychiatry* 1994; 150 (Suppl. 4):1–26.

American Psychiatric Association; "Practice guideline for the treatment of patients with bipolar disorder." *American Journal of Psychiatry* 1994; 151 (Suppl. 12):1–35.

"An Alternative Mood Booster." *Health* 1996 Nov 11; 10(7).

Anderson J., Deskins B.; *The Nutrition Bible*. New York: William Morrow & Company, 1995.

Baureithel K. H., Buter K. B., Engesser A., Burkard W., Schaffner W.; "Inhibition of benzodiazepine binding *in vitro* by amentoflavone, a constituent of various species of Hypericum." *Pharm Acta Helv* 1997 June; 72(3):153–7.

Beckstrom-Sternberg S., Duke J. A.; "Chemicals and their biological activities in: Hypericum perforatum L. (Clusiaceae)-Common St. John's Wort, Hypericum, Klamath Weed." Phytochemical Database-USDA-ARS-NGRL.

Berger P. A., Nemeroff C. B.; "Opiod peptides in affective disorders." *Psychopharmacology: The Third Generation of Progress*. Meltzer H. Y., ed. New York: Raven Press 1987, 637–646.

Berghoefer R., Hoelzl J.; "Biflavonoids in Hypericum perforatum, Part 1. Isolation of 13, II8-biapigenin." *Planta Medica* 53:216–7.

Bladt S., Wagner H.; "Inhibition of MAO by fractions and constituents of Hypericum extract." *Journal of Geriatric Psychiatry and Neurology* 1994 October; 7 Suppl 1:S57–9.

Bol'shakova I. V., Lozovskaia E. L., Sapezhinskii I. I.; "Antioxidant properties of a series of extracts from medicinal plants." [Russian; English abstract] *Biofizika* 1997 March–April; 42(2):480–3.

Bol'shakova I. V., Lozovskaia E. L., Sapezhinskii I. I.; "Photosensitizing and photoprotective properties of extracts from groups of medicinal plants." [Russian; English abstract] *Biofizika* 1997 July–August; 42(4):926–32.

Boxer A., Back P.; *The Herb Book*. London: Peerage Books, 1989.

Bremness L.; *The Complete Book of Herbs: A Practical Guide to Growing and Using Herbs*. Viking Studio Books, 1988.

Brockmoller J., Reum T., Bauer S., Kerb R., Hubner W. D., Roots I.; "Hypericin and pseudohypericin: pharmacokinetics and effects on photosensitivity in humans." *Pharmacopsychiatry* 1997 September; 30 Suppl 2:94–101.

Brooklyn Botanic Garden; Metropolitan Plant Encyclopedia @*http://www.bbg.org*.

Brousseau California Flora collection @*http://elib.cs.berkeley.edu*.

Bruneton, J.; *Pharmacognosy, Phytochemistry, Medicinal Plants*. Andover, England: Intercept, Ltd., 1995.

Buchanan, R., ed.; *Taylor's Guide to Herbs*. Boston: Houghton Mifflin, 1995.

Bunney W. E., Davis J. M.; "Norepinephrine in depressive reactions: A review." *Archives of General Psychiatry* 1965; 13A:483–94 1965.

Burke M. J., Silkey B., Preskorn S. H.; "Pharmacoeconomic considerations when evaluating treatment options for major depressive disorder." *Journal of Clinical Psychiatry* 1994; 55(suppl. A):42–52.

Butterweck V., Wall A., Lieflander-Wulf U., Winterhoff H., Nahrstedt A.; "Effects of the total extract and fractions of Hypericum perforatum in animal assays for antidepressant activity." *Pharmacopsychiatry* 1997 September; 30 Suppl 2: 117–24.

Centers for Disease Control and Prevention, National Center for Health Statistics.

Charney D. S., Menkes D. B., Heninger G. R.; "Receptor sensitivity and the mechanism of action of antidepressant treatment: Implications for the etiology and therapy of depression." *Archives of General Psychiatry* 1981; 38:1160–80.

Clarkson, R. E.; *The Golden Age of Herbs and Herbalists.* New York: Dover Publications, 1972.

Coccaro E. F., Silverman J. M., Klar H. M., Horwath T. B., Siever L. J.; "Familial correlates of reduced central serotonergic system function in patients with personality disorders." *Archives of General Psychiatry* 1994; 51:318–24.

Consumer Guide, in consultation with the American Association of Naturopathic Physicians; *Alternative Medicine.* Lincolnwood, IL: Publications International Ltd., 1997.

Cook N., Samman S.; "Flavonoids—Chemistry, metabolism, cardioprotective effects, and dietary sources." *Journal of Nutritional Biochemistry* 1996; 7:66–76.

Coon N.; *The Dictionary of Useful Plants.* Emmaus, PA: Rodale Press, 1974.

Cooper J. R., Bloom F. E., Roth R. H.; *The Biochemical Basis of Neuropharmacology.* New York: Oxford University Press, 1991.

Cott J.; "NCDEU Update: Natural product formulations available in Europe for psychotropic indications." *Psychopharmacology Bulletin* 1995; 31(4):745–51.

Cott J. M.; "In vitro receptor binding and enzyme inhibition by Hypericum perforatum extract." *Pharmacopsychiatry* 1997 September; 30 Suppl 2:108–12.

Cracchiolo C.; FAQ on St. Johns Wort (Hypericum perforatum and Hypericum augustofolia) @*http://www.primenet.com/~camilla/STJOHNS.FAQ.*

Crellin J. K., Philpott J.; *Herbal Medicine Past and Present, Volume II: A Reference Guide to Medicinal Plants.* Durham, NC: Duke University Press, 1990.

Culpeper N.; *Culpeper's Complete Herbal: Consisting of a Comprehensive Description of Nearly All Herbs With Their*

Medicinal Properties and Directions for Compound. London: Foulsham & Co. Ltd., 1995.

Cummings S., Ullman D.; *Everybody's Guide to Homeopathic Medicines*. New York: G. P. Putnam's Sons, 1991.

Czekalla J., Gastpar M., Hubner W. D., Jager D.; "The effect of Hypericum extract on cardiac conduction as seen in the electrocardiogram compared to that of imipramine." *Pharmacopsychiatry* 1997 September; 30 Suppl 2:86–8.

Davidov M. I., Goriunov V. G., Kubarikov P. G.; "Phytoperfusion of the bladder after adenomectomy." [Russian; English abstract] *Urologiia I Nefrologiia* 1995 September–October; (5):19–20.

Davidson J. R. T., Miller R. D., Turnbull C. D., Sullivan J. L.; "Atypical depression." *Archives of General Psychiatry* 1982; 39:527–34.

De Smet P. A., Nolen W. A.; "St. John's Wort as an antidepressant." *British Medical Journal* 1996 August 3; 313(7052): 241–2.

Depression Guideline Panel (Clinical Practice Guideline No. 5); "Depression in primary care: Vol. 2. Treatment of major depression" *AHCPR Publication No. 93-0551*; Rockville, MD: U.S. Department of Health and Human Services, Agency for Health Care Policy and Research.

Depue R. A., Spoont M. R.; "Conceptualizing a serotonin trait as a behavioral dimension of constraint." Mann J. L., Stanley M., eds. *Psychobiology of Suicidal Behavior*. New York: New York Academy of Sciences, 1986, 47–62.

Derbentseva N. A.; "Actions of tannins from Hypericum perforatum L on the influenza virus." *Mikrobial* 1972 311(6): 768–72.

Dimpfel W., Hofmann R.; "Pharmacodynamic effects of St. John's Wort on rat intracerebral field potentials." *European*

Journal of Medical Research 1995 December 18; 1(3):157–67.

Diwu Z.; "Novel therapeutic and diagnostic applications of hypocrellins and hypericins." *Photochemistry-Photobiology* 1995 June; 61(6):529–39.

Dobson K. S.; "A meta-analysis of the efficacy of cognitive therapy for depression." *Journal of Consulting Clinical Psychiatry* 1989.

Dorossiev I.; "Determination of flavonoids in Hypericum perforatum." *Phytochemistry* 1985; 40:585–6.

Duke J. A.; *The Green Pharmacy*. Emmaus, PA: Rodale Press, 1997.

Elliott J. M.; "Peripheral markers in affective disorders" in *Biological Aspects of Affective Disorders*. Horton R. W., Katona C. L. E., eds. San Diego: Academic Press, 1991, 96–144.

Ernst E.; "St. John's Wort, an antidepressive? A systematic criteria-based review." *Phytomedicine* 1995 2(1):67–71.

Ernst E.; "St. John's Wort as antidepressive therapy." [German; English abstract] *Fortschritte Der Medizin* 1995 September 10; 113(25):354–5.

Evstifeeva T. A., Sibiriak S. V.; "The immunotropic properties of biologically active products obtained from Klamath weed (Hypericum perforatum L.)." [Russian; English abstract] *Eksperimentalnaia I Klinicheskaia Farmakologiia* 1996 January–February; 59(1):51–4.

Frank E., Karp J. F., Rush A. J.; "Efficacy of treatments for major depression." *Psychopharmacology Bulletin* 1993; 29:457–75.

Garland S.; *Growing and Using Culinary, Aromatic, Cosmetic and Medicinal Plants*. New York: Readers Digest, 1993.

Gerard J.; *The Herbal or General History of Plants*. New York: Dover Publications, 1975.

Gillespie R. D.; "The clinical differentiation of types of depression." *Guy's Hospital Reports* 1929; 79:306–44.

Ginzberg E., Dutka A.; *The Financing of Biomedical Research*. Baltimore: Johns Hopkins University Press, 1989.

Gold P. W., Goodwin F. K., Chrousos G. P.; "Clinical and biochemical manifestations of depression, part 2. Relation to the neurobiology of stress." *New England Journal of Medicine* 1988; 319:413–20.

Goldberg I.; Dr. Ivan's Depression Central @ *http://www.psycom.net/depression.central.html*.

Golsch S., Vocks E., Rakoski J., Brockow K., Ring J.; "Reversible increase in photosensitivity to UV-B caused by St. John's Wort extract." [German; English abstract] *Hautarzt* 1997 April 48(4):249–52.

Goodwin F. K., Jamison K. R.; *Manic-Depressive Illness*. New York: Oxford University Press, 1990.

Grieve M.; *A Modern Herbal: The medical, culinary, cosmetic and economic properties, cultivation and folklore of herbs, grasses, fungi, shrubs, and trees with all their modern scientific uses*. New York: Penguin Books, 1988.

Hänsgen K. D., Vesper J., Ploch M.; "Multicenter double-blind study examining the antidepressant effectiveness of the Hypericum extract LI-160." *Journal of Geriatric Psychiatry and Neurology* 1994 October; 7 Suppl. 1:S15–8.

Harborne J. B., Mabry T. J. editors; *The Flavonoids: Advances in Research*. New York: Chapman and Hall, 1982.

Harrer G., Hübner W. D., Podzuweit H.; "Effectiveness and tolerance of the Hypericum extract LI-160 compared to maprotiline: a multicenter double-blind study." *Journal of Ger-*

iatric Psychiatry and Neurology 1994 October; 7 Suppl. 1: S24–8.

Harrer G., Schultz.; "Clinical investigation of the antidepressant effectiveness of Hypericum." *Journal of Geriatric Psychiatry and Neurology* 1994 October; 7 Suppl. 1:S6–8.

Harrer G., Sommer H.; "Treatment of mild/moderate depressions with Hypericum."*Phytomedicine* 1994 1:3–8.

Haughton C.; "Hypericum Perforatum." Health Centre Herb Monographs 1997 September 26.

Hobbs C.; "St. John's Wort: A Review." *HerbalGram* Fall 1988/Winter 1989; 18/19:24–33.

Hoffman, D.; *The New Holistic Herbal*, 3rd Edition. Rockport, MA: Element Books, 1999.

Hollon S. D., DeRubeis R. J., Evans M. D., Wiemer M. J., Garvey M. J., Grover W. M., Tuason V. B.; "Cognitive-therapy and pharmacotherapy for depression: Singly and in Combination." *Archives of General Psychiatry* 1992; 49:774–81.

Holzl J., Ostrowski E.; "Analysis of the essential compounds of Hypericum perforatum." *Planta Medica*: 531.

Horne J. A.; "Human sleep loss and behavior implications for the prefrontal cortex and psychiatric disorder." *British Journal of Psychiatry* 1991; 30:283–304.

Howland R. H., Thase M. E.; "A comprehensive review of cyclothymic disorder." *Journal of Nervous and Mental Disease* 1993; 181:485–93.

Howland R. H., Thase M. E.; "Biological studies of Dysthymia." *Biological Psychiatry* 1991; 30:283–304.

Hsaio J. K., Agren H., Bartko J. J., Rudorfer M. V., Linnoila M., Potter W. Z.; "Monoamine neurotransmitter interactions and the prediction of antidepressant response." *Archives of General Psychiatry* 1987; 44:1078–1083.

Hübner W. D., Lande S., Podzuweit H.; "Hypericum treatment of mild depression with somatic symptoms." *Journal of Geriatric Psychiatry and Neurology* 1994 October; 7 Suppl. 1:S15–8.

Huston P. E., Locher L. M.; "Manic-depressive psychosis: course when treated and untreated with electric shock." *Archives of Neurology and Psychiatry* 1948; 50:37–48.

James, J. S.; "Hypericum: Common herb shows antiretroviral activity. From Medical Virology Conference." *AIDS Treatment News* 1988 August 26; (63).

Jarrett R. B.; "Psycho-social aspects of depression and the role of psychotherapy." *Journal of Clinical Psychiatry* 1990; 51: 26–35.

Johnson D., Ksciuk H., Woelk H., Sauerwein-Giese E., Frauendorf A.; "Effects of Hypericum extract LI-160 compared with maprotiline on resting EEG and evoked potentials in 24 volunteers." *Journal of Geriatric Psychiatry and Neurology* 1994 October; 7 Suppl. 1:S44–6.

Kartnig T., Gobel I., Heydel B.; "Production of hypericin, pseudohypericin and flavonoids in cell cultures of various Hypericum species and their chemotypes." *Planta Medica* 1996 February; 62(1):51–3.

Kasper S.; "Treatment of seasonal affective disorder (SAD) with Hypericum extract." *Pharmacopsychiatry* 1997 September; 30 Suppl. 2:89–93.

Keller M. B., Shapiro R. W.; " 'Double-Depression': Superimposition of acute depressive episodes on chronic depressive disorders." *American Journal of Psychiatry* 1982; 139:438–42.

Kerb R., Brockmoller J., Staffeldt B., Ploch M., Roots I.;

"Single-dose and steady-state pharmacokinetics of hypericin and pseudohypericin." *Antimicrobial Agents and Chemotherapy* 1996 September; 40(9):2087–93.

Keville, K.; *Herbs: An Illustrated Encyclopedia: A Complete Culinary, Cosmetic, Medicinal and Ornamental Guide.* New York: Friedman/Fairfax Publishers, 1994.

Kinghorn D. A, Balandrin M. F., editors; *Human Medicinal Agents from Plants.* Washington, DC: American Chemical Society, 1993.

Kocsis J. H.; "DSM-IV 'major depression': Are more stringent criteria needed?" *Depression* 1993; 1:24–28.

Kraepelin E.; *Manic Depressive Insanity and Paranoia.* Edinburgh: Livingstone; 1921.

Kramer, P. D.; *Listening to Prozac: A Psychiatrist Explores Antidepressant Drugs and the Remaking of the Self.* New York: Viking, 1993.

Kress, H.; *http://www.sunsite.unc.edu.*

Krylov A. A., Ibatov A. N.; "The use of an infusion of St. John's Wort in the combined treatment of alcoholics with peptic ulcer and chronic gastritis." *Likarska Sprava* 1993 February–March; (2–3):146–8.

Kumper H.; "Hypericum poisoning in sheep." *Tierarztliche Praxis* 1989; 17(3):257–61.

Kupfer D. J.; "Long-term treatment of depression." *Journal of Clinical Psychiatry* 1991; 52:28–42.

Kupfer D. J., Thase M. E.; "Validity of major depression: a psychobiological perspective." *Diagnostic and Classification in Psychiatry: A critical appraisal of DSM-III.* Tischler G. M., ed. New York: Cambridge University Press, 1987, 32–60.

Lavie G.; "Hypericin as an inactivation of infectious viruses in blood components." *Transfusion* 1995 May; 35(5):392–400.

Lima P.; *The Harrowsmith Illustrated Book of Herbs*. New York/Ontario: Camden House, 1986.

Linde K., Ramirez G., Mulrow C. D., Pauls A., Weidenhammer W., Melchart D.; "St. John's Wort for depression—an overview and meta-analysis of randomized clinical trials." *British Medical Journal* 1996 August 3; 313(7052):253–8. Also comment in *British Medical Journal* 1996 November 9; 313(7066):1204–5.

Linnoila V. M., Virkkunen M.; "Aggression suicidality and serotonin." *Journal of Clinical Psychiatry* 1992; 53:46–51.

Lucas R. M.; *Nature's Medicines: The folklore, romance and value of herbal remedies*. West Nyack, NY: Parker Publishing Co., 1966.

Lust J.; *The Herb Book*. New York: Bantam Books, 1974.

Malone K., Mann J. J.; "Serotonin and major depression." *Biology of Depressive Disorders: Part A*. Mann J. J., Kupfer D. J., eds.; New York: Plenum Press, 1993, 29–49.

Marcin M. M.; *The Herbal Tea Garden: Planning, planting, harvesting & brewing*. Pownal, VT: Storey Communications, 1993.

Martin L. C.; *Garden Flower Folklore*. Old Saybrook, CT: The Globe Pequot Press, 1987.

Martinez B., Kasper S., Ruhrmann B., Möller H. J.; "Hypericum in the treatment of seasonal affective disorder." *Journal of Geriatric Psychiatry and Neurology* 1994 October; 7 Suppl. 1:S29–33.

McCarley R. W.; "REM sleep and depression: Common neurobiological control mechanisms." *American Journal of Psychiatry* 1982: 139:565–570.

The Medical Advisor: The Complete Guide to Alternative and Conventional Treatments. New York: Time Life.

Melzer R., Fricke U., Hölzl J.; "Vasoactive properties of procyanidins from Hypericum perforatum L in isolated porcine coronary arteries." *Arzneimittelforschung* 1991 May; 41(5): 481–3.

Meruelo D., Lavie G., Lavie D.; "Therapeutic agents with dramatic antiretroviral activity and little toxicity at effective doses: aromatic polycyclic diones hypericin and pseudohypericin." Proceedings of the National Academy of Sciences of the United States 1988 July; 85(14):5230–4.

Mintz J., Mintz L. I., Arruda M. J., Hwang S. S.; "Treatments of depression and the functional capacity to work." *Archives of General Psychiatry* 1992; 49:761–8.

Monk T. H.; "Biological rhythms and depressive disorders." *Biology of Depressive Disorders: Part A.* Mann J. J., Kupfer D. J., eds.; New York: Plenum Press, 1993, 109–122.

Muldner H., Zoller, M.; "Antidepressive effect of a Hypericum extract standardized to an active hypericine complex— biochemical and clinical studies." *Arzneimittelforschung* 1984; 34(8):918–20.

Muller W. E., Rolli M., Schafer C., Hafner U.; "Effects of Hypericum extract (LI-160) in biochemical models of antidepressant activity." *Pharmacopsychiatry* 1997 September; 30 Suppl. 2:102–7.

Muller W. E., Rossol R.; "Effects of Hypericum extract on the expression of serotonin receptors." *Journal of Geriatric Psychiatry and Neurology* 1994 October; 7 Suppl. 1:S63–4.

Murray M.; *The Healing Power of Herbs, revised and expanded, 2nd edition.* Rocklin, CA: Prima Publishing, 1995.

Nahrstedt A., Butterweck V.; "Biologically active and other chemical constituents of the herb of Hypericum perforatum

L." *Pharmacopsychiatry* 1997 September; 30 Suppl. 2:129–34.

Nemeroff C. B.; "New vistas in neuropeptide research in neuropsychiatry: Focus on corticotropin-releasing factor." *Neuropsychopharmacology* 1992; 6:69–75.

Norden, M.; *Beyond Prozac: Brain-Toxic Lifestyles, Natural Antidotes & New Generation Antidepressants.* New York: Regan Books, 1996.

Nordfors M., Hartvig P.; "St. John's Wort against depression in favour again." [Swedish; English abstract] *Lakartidningen* 1997 June 18; 94(25):2365–67.

Ody, Penelope. *The Complete Medicinal Herbal.* New York: Dorling Kindersley, 1993.

Okie S.; "Saint John's Wort may ease mild to moderate depression." *The Washington Post* 1997, October 14; z12.

Okpanyi S. N., Lidzba H., Scholl B. C., Mittenburger H. G.; "Genotoxicity of a standardized Hypericum extract." [German; English abstract] *Arzneimittelforschung* 1990; 40(8): 851–5.

Okpanyi S. N., Weischer M. L.; "Experimental animal studies of the psychotropic activity of a Hypericum Extract." [German; English abstract] *Arzneimittelforschung* 1987; 37(1): 10–3.

Oren D. A., Rosenthal N. E.; "Seasonal Affective Disorders." *Handbook of Affective Disorders, 2nd ed.* Paykel P. S., ed.; New York: Guilford Press, 1992.

Ozturk Y.; "Testing the antidepressant effects of Hypericum species on animal models." *Pharmacopsychiatry* 1997 September; 30 Suppl. 2:125–8.

Panos M., Heimlich J.; *Homeopathic Remedies at Home.* G. P. Putnam's Sons, 1980.

Payk T. R.; "Treatment of depression." *Journal of Geriatric Psychiatry and Neurology* 1994 October; 7 Suppl.. 1:S3–5.

Perovic S., Muller W. E.; "Pharmacological profile of Hypericum extract. Effect on serotonin uptake by postsynaptic receptors." *Arzneimittelforschung* 1995 November; 45(11): 1145–8.

Persons J. B., Thase M. E., Crits-Christoph P.; "The role of psychotherapy in the treatment of depression." *s* 1996; 53: 283–90.

Piperopoulos G., Lotz R., Wixforth A., Schmierer T., Zeller K. P.; "Determination of naphthodianthrones in plant extracts from Hypericum perforatum L. by liquid chromatography-electrospray mass spectrometry." *Journal of Chromatography B Biomed Sci Appl* 1997 August 1; 695(2):309–16.

Post R. M.; "Transduction of psychosocial stress into the neurobiology of recurrent affective disorder." *American Journal of Psychiatry* 1992; 149:999–1010.

Preskorn S. H., Burke M.; "Somatic therapy for major depressive disorder: Selection of an antidepressant." *Journal of Clinical Psychiatry* 1992; 53(suppl. 9):5, 18.

Prien R. F., Kocsis J. H.; "Long-term treatment of mood disorder." *Psychopharmacology: The Fourth Generation of Progress*. Bloom F. E., Kupfer D. J., eds; New York: Raven Press, 1995, 1067–1079.

Prien R. F., Kupfer D. J.; "Continuation drug therapy for major depressive episodes: How long should it be maintained?" *American Journal of Psychiatry* 1986; 143:18–23.

Rampes H., "Hypericum, an over the counter antidepressant?" *Journal of Psychopharmacology* (Oxf) 1997; 11(2): 191.

Rath G., Potterat O., Mavi S., Hostettmann K.; "Xanthones

from Hypericum roeperanum." *Phytochemistry* 1996 September; 43(2):513–20.

Reiger D., Hirschfield R., Goodwin F., Burke J. Lazar J., Judd L.; "The NIMH Depression, Awareness, Recognition, and Treatment Program: Structure, aims, and scientific basis." *American Journal of Psychiatry* 1988; 145:1351–57.

Reiger D. A., Narrow W. E., Rae D. S., Manderscheid R. W., Locke B. Z., Goodwin F. K.; "The *defacto* U.S. mental and addictive disorder service system. Epidemiological catchment area prospective 1-year prevalence rates of disorders and services." *Archives of General Psychiatry* 1993; 50:85–94.

Rivera D., Obon C.; "The ethnopharmacology of Madeira and Porto Santo Islands, a review." *Journal of Ethnopharmacology* 1995 May; 46(2):73–93.

Rocha L., Marston A., Potterat O., Kaplan M.A., Stoeckli-Evans H., Hostettmann K.; "Antibacterial phloroglucinols and flavonoids from Hypericum brasiliense." *Phytochemistry* 1995 November; 40(5):1447–52.

Sandler M., Ruthven C. R., Goodwin B. L., Coppen A.; "Decreased cerebrospinal fluid concentration of free phenylacetic acid in depressive illness." *Clinica Chimica Acta* 1979; 93: 169–171.

Schmidt U., Sommer H.; "St. John's Wort extract in the ambulatory therapy of depression" *Fortschritte Der Medizin* 1993 July 10; 111(19):339–42.

Schulz H., Jobert M.; "Effects of Hypericum extract on the sleep EEG in older volunteers." *Journal of Geriatric Psychiatry and Neurology* 1994 October; 7 Suppl 1:S39–43.

Sclar D. A., Robinson L. M., Skaer T. L., Legg R. F., Nemec N. L., Galin R. S., Hughes T. E., Bueschling D. P.; "Antidepressant pharmacotherapy: Economic outcomes in a health maintenance organization." *Clinical Therapeutics* 1994; 16: 715–730.

"The Secrets of Saint John's Wort." *Prevention* 1997 February 1; 49(2).

Siever L. J., Davis K. L.; "A psychobiological perspective on personality disorders." *American Journal of Psychiatry* 1991; 148(12); 1647–1658.

Smyshliaeva A. V., Kudriashov I. B.; "The modification of a radiation lesion in animals with an aqueous extract of Hypericum perforatum L." *Nauchnye Doklady Vysshei Shkoly. Biologicheskie Nauki* 1992; (4):7–9.

Smyshliaeva A. V., Nguyen L. H., Kudriashov I. B.; "The modification of a radiation lesion in animals with an aqueous extract of Hypericum perforatum L." *Nauchnye Doklady Vysshei Shkoly. Biologicheskie Nauki* 1992; (4):9–13.

Sommer H., Harrer G.; "Placebo-controlled double-blind study examining the effectiveness of an Hypericum preparation in 105 mildly depressed patients." *Journal of Geriatric Psychiatry and Neurology* 1994 October; 7 Suppl 1:S9–11.

Song F., Freemantle N., Sheldon T. A.; "Selective serotonin reuptake inhibitors: meta-analysis of efficacy and acceptability." *British Journal of Medicine* 1993; 306:683–687.

"St. John's Wort." *Med Lett Drugs Ther* 1997 November 21; 39(1014):107–8.

Staffeldt B., Kerb R., Brockmoller J., Ploch M., Roots I.; "Pharmacokinetics of hypericin and pseudohypericin after oral intake of the Hypericum perforatum extract LI-160 in healthy volunteers." *Journal of Geriatric Psychiatry and Neurology* 1994 October; 7 Suppl 1:S47–53.

Steinbeck-Klose A., Wernet P.; "Successful long-term treatment over 40 months of HIV patients with intravenous hypericin." International Conference on AIDS 1993 June 6–11; 9(1):470.

Takahashi J., Nakanishi S., Kobayashi E., Nakano H., Suzuki

K., Tamaoki T.; ''Hypericin and pseudohypericin specifically inhibit protein kinase C: possible relation to their retroviral activity.'' *Biochemical and Biophysical Research Communications* 1989 December 29, 165(3):1207–12.

Tammaro F., Xepapdakis G.; ''Plants used in phytotherapy, cosmetics and dyeing in the Pramanda district (Esprius, North-West Greece).'' *Journal of Ethnopharmacology* 1986 June; 16(2–3): 167–74.

Taylor R. S., Manandhar N. P., Hudson J. B., Towers G. H.; ''Antiviral activities of Nepalese medicinal plants.'' *Journal of Ethnopharmacology* 1996 July 5; 52(3):157–63.

Teufel-Mayer R., Gleitz J.; ''Effects of long-term administration of Hypericum extracts on the affinity and density of the central serotonergic 5-HT1 A and 5-HT2 A receptors.'' *Pharmacopsychiatry* 1997 September; 30 Suppl 2:113–6.

Thase M. E.; ''Long term treatments of recurrent depressive disorders.'' *Journal of Clinical Psychiatry* 1992; 53(suppl. 8): 33–44.

Thase M. E.; ''Maintenance treatments of recurrent affective disorder.'' *Current Opinion in Psychiatry* 1993; 6:16–21.

Thase M. E.; ''Reeducative psychotherapy.'' *Treatments of psychiatric disorders: DSM-IV edition.* Gabbard G., ed. Washington, DC: American Psychiatric Press, 1995, 1169–1204.

Thase M. E., Carpenter L., Kupfer D. J., Frank E.; Clinical significance of reversed vegetative sub-types of recurrent major depression.'' *Psychopharmacology Bulletin* 1991; 27:17–22.

Thase M. E., Daley D. C.; ''Understanding Depression and Addiction.'' *Dual Diagnostic Series*, Center City, MN: Hazelden Educational Materials, 1994.

Thase M. E., Frank E., Kupfer D. J.; ''Biological processes in major depression.'' *Handbook of Depression: Treatment, As-*

sessment, Research. Beckham E. E., Leber W. R., eds. Homewood, IL: Dorsey Press, 1985, 816–913.

Thase M. E., Hersen M., Bellack A. S., Himmelhoch J. M., Kupfer D. J. "Validation of a Hamilton subscale for endogenomorphic depression." *Journal of Affective Disorders* 1983; 5:267–278.

Thase M. E., Himmelhoch J. M.; "On the Amish study." *American Journal of Psychiatry* 1983; 140:1263–1264.

Thase, M. E., Himmelhoch J. M., Mallinger A. G., Jarret D. B., Kupfer D. J.; "Sleep EEG and DST findings in anergic bipolar depression." *American Journal of Psychiatry* 1989; 146:329–33.

Thase, M. E., Howland R.; "Refractory depression: Relevance of psychosocial factors and therapies." *Psychiatric Annals* 1994; 24:232–40.

Thase M. E., Howland R. H.; "Biological Processes in Depression: An Updated Review and Integration." *Handbook of Depression, 2nd edition*. Beckman E. E., Leber W. R., eds.; New York: Guilford, 1995, 213–279.

Thase, M. E., Kupfer D. J.; "Recent Developments in the Pharmacotherapy of Mood Disorders." *Journal of Consulting and Clinical Psychology* 1996; 64(4):646–59.

Thase M. E., Rush A. J.; "Treatment resistant depression." *Psychopharmacology: The Fourth Generation of Progress*. New York: Raven Press, 1995, 1081–97.

Thase M. E., Simons A. D., Reynolds C. F.; "Psychobiological correlates of poor response to cognitive behavior therapy: Potential indications for antidepressant pharmacotherapy." *Psychopharmacology* 1993; 29:293–301.

Thiede H. M., Walper A.; "Inhibition of MAO and COMT by Hypericum extracts and hypericin." *Journal of Geriatric Psychiatry and Neurology* 1994 October; 7 Suppl 1:S54–6.

Thiele B., Brink I., Ploch M.; "Modulation of cytokine expression by Hypericum extract." [German; English translation] *Journal of Geriatric Psychiatry and Neurology* 1994 October; 7 Suppl 1:S60–2.

Thomas C., MacGill R. S., Neill P., Pardini R. S.; "The *in vitro* and *in vivo* photoinduced antineoplastic activity of hypericin." Proceedings: Annual Meeting of the American Association for Cancer Research 1992; 33:A2989.

Tsuang M. T., Faraone S. V.; *The Genetics of Mood Disorders*. Baltimore: Johns Hopkins University Press, 1990.

Tyler, V. E.; *Herbs of Choice: The Therapeutic Use of Phytomedicinals*. New York: Haworth Press, 1994.

Tyler, V. E.; *The Honest Herbal*. New York: Haworth Press, 1994.

Tyler, V. E., Brady, L. R., Robbers, J. E.; *Pharmacognosy, 9th Edition*. Philadelphia: Lea & Febiger, 1988.

USDA-ARS-GRIN database.

Vickery R.; *A Dictionary of Plant Lore*. New York: Oxford University Press, 1995.

Volz H. P.; "Controlled clinical trials of Hypericum extracts in depressed patients—an overview." *Pharmacopsychiatry* 1997 September; 30 Suppl 2:72–6.

Von Korff M., Ormel J., Katon W., Lin E. H. B.; "Disability and depression among utilizers of health care. A longitudinal analysis." *Archives of General Psychiatry* 1992; 49:91–100.

Vonsover A., Steibeck K. A., Rudich C., Mazur Y., Lavie D., Mandel M., Lavie G.; "HIV-1 virus load in the serum of AIDS patients undergoing long term therapy with hypericin." International Conference on AIDS; 1996 July 7–12; 11(1):120.

Vorbach E. U., Arnoldt K. H., Hubner W. D.; "Efficacy and

tolerability of St. John's Wort extract LI 160 versus imipramine in patients with severe depressive episodes according to ICD-10." *Pharmacopsychiatry* 1997 September; 30 Suppl 2: 81–5.

Vorbach E. U., Hubner W. D., Arnoldt K. H.; "Effectiveness and tolerance of the Hypericum extract LI 160 in comparison with imipramine: randomized double-blind study with 135 outpatients." *Journal of Geriatric Psychiatry and Neurology* 1994 October; 7 Suppl 1:S19–23.

Wagner H., Bladt S.; "Pharmaceutical quality of Hypericum extracts." *Journal of Geriatric Psychiatry and Neurology* 1994 October; 7 Suppl 1:S65–8.

Wehr T. A., Rosenthal N. E.; "Seasonality of affective disorder." *American Journal of Psychiatry* 1989; 146:829–839.

Weiss J. M.; "Stress-induced depression: Critical neurochemical and electrophysiological changes." *Neurobiology of Learning Emotion and Affect.* Madden J., ed. New York: Raven Press, 1991, 123–154.

Wells K. B., Katon W., Rogers B., Camp P.; "Use of minor tranquilizers and antidepressant medications by depressed outpatients: Results from the medical outcomes study." *American Journal of Psychiatry* 1994; 151:694–700.

Wheatley D.; "LI 160, an extract of St. John's Wort, versus amitriptyline in mildly to moderately depressed outpatients—a controlled 6-week clinical trial." *Pharmacopsychiatry* 1997 September; 30 Suppl 2:77–80.

Wichtl M.; *Herbal Drugs and Phytopharmaceuticals.* N. Bisset, translator. Boca Raton: CRC Press, 1994.

Winter R.; *Nutraceuticals.* New York: Crown Trade Paperbacks, 1995.

Witte B., Harrer G., Kaptan T., Podzuweit H., Schmidt U.; "Treatment of depressive symptoms with a high concentration

Hypericum preparation. A multicenter placebo-controlled double-blind study.'' [German; English abstract] *Fortschritte Der Medizin* 1995 October 10; 113(28):404–8.

Woelk H., Burkard G., Grunwald J.; ''Benefits and risks of the Hypericum extract LI-160: drug monitoring study with 3250 patients.'' *Journal of Geriatric Psychiatry and Neurology* 1994 October; 7 Suppl 1:S34–8.

Wood M.; *The Book of Herbal Wisdom: Using plants as medicines.* Berkley, CA: North Atlantic Books, 1997.

Zornberg G. L., Pope H. G.; ''Treatment of depression in bipolar disorder: New directions for research.'' *Journal of Clinical Psychopharmacology* 1993; 13:397–408.

Index